CLINICAL INVESTIGATIONS

CLINICAL INVESTIGATIONS

Allen Bernard Shaw

MD, FRCP
Consultant Physician to the Bradford Hospitals;
Visiting Lecturer to the University of Bradford
West Yorkshire, England

Baillière Tindall
LONDON PHILADELPHIA TORONTO MEXICO CITY
RIO DE JANEIRO SYDNEY TOKYO HONG KONG

Baillière Tindall   1 St Anne's Road
W. B. Saunders   Eastbourne, East Sussex BN21 3UN, England

West Washington Square
Philadelphia, PA 19105, USA

1 Goldthorne Avenue
Toronto, Ontario M8Z 5T9, Canada

Apartado 26370 — Cedro 512
Mexico 4, DF Mexico

Rua Evaristo da Veiga 55, 20° andar
Rio de Janeiro — RJ, Brazil

ABP Australia Ltd, 44–50 Waterloo Road
North Ryde, NSW 2113, Australia

Ichibancho Central Building, 22–1 Ichibancho
Chiyoda-ku, Tokyo 102, Japan

10/fl, Inter-Continental Plaza, 94 Granville Road
Tsim Sha Tsui East, Kowloon, Hong Kong

© 1984 Baillière Tindall

First published 1984

Typeset by Photographics, Honiton, Devon
Printed and bound in Great Britain by
Richard Clay (the Chaucer Press) Ltd
Bungay, Suffolk

British Library Cataloguing in Publication Data

Shaw, Allen Bernard
    Clinical investigations.
    1.   Diagnosis
    I.   Title
    616.07'5   RC71

    ISBN   0–7020–1057–X

CONTENTS

PREFACE

The compilation of these notes has been prompted by my frequent failure to fully understand the results of laboratory tests that I had personally requested. My aim has been to answer some of the many questions raised by such results and to provide a brief guide to further investigation. The selection of material, therefore, has been guided by my own clinical experience, in a district general hospital in the United Kingdom, keeping especially in mind the needs of a house officer looking at the evening laboratory reports. It is arguable that a single clinician cannot deal with so many diverse disciplines. My excuse and hope is that what has been lost in authority has been gained in immediate clinical relevance.

I am indebted to several colleagues for advice, notably Dr A. M. Davison, Dr. W. E. Edgar, Dr P. J. Hollins, Dr O. J. Follows, Dr A. T. Howarth, Dr M. R. Jeffrey, Dr P. C. Reynell, Dr D. R. Smith, Professor R. L. Turner and Dr R. L. Woodhead. I am also indebted to Mrs J. Verity for her careful typing, Mr Graham Smith of Baillière Tindall for his wise guidance, and above all to my wife for her extreme patience and constant encouragement.

Allen Bernard Shaw

INTRODUCTION

This book is divided into chapters, along the lines of a conventional medical text. Each chapter begins with a brief introduction, dealing mainly with the most relevant physiology. Commonly used tests are then discussed, with emphasis on tests reported in figures or simple statements. Biochemistry, haematology and bacteriology predominate, but the possibilities of important imaging techniques have been indicated. Some basic electrocardiography has been included, with the nocturnal labours of resident staff in mind. The chapters conclude with discussion of the investigation of common clinical problems.

With each test a range of normal values in adults is given in Système International (SI) units. Where relevant, the figures for children, pregnancy and old age follow. The term neonate indicates an age below one month, and infancy, below two years. It is up to the reader to decide when old age begins. Any normal value given in this book should be disregarded if those issued by the local laboratory are different. The specimen required is usually clotted blood, which should be taken to the laboratory as soon as possible, unless otherwise stated. Again, this may vary with the method of measurement used locally. The causes of abnormal values are given, but the lists exclude conditions thought to be sufficiently rare. The clinical effects of biochemical changes are mentioned where appropriate. An outline of the procedure for some clinical tests is given, as incorrect methods cause misleading results.

This is a brief guide, not a comprehensive text. Some useful further sources of information are given in Appendix I. Apart from these, I would recommend that a search for information start with a general textbook and proceed through specialized texts, review articles and, finally, original papers. This search will be shortened by personal contact with people working in the particular field.

LIST OF ABBREVIATIONS

ACE	Angiotensin converting enzyme	**Ccr**	Creatinine clearance
ACTH	Adrenocorticotrophic hormone (corticotrophin)	**CFT**	Complement fixation test
		CMI	Cell-mediated immunity
ADH	Antidiuretic hormone (vasopressin)	**CML**	Chronic myeloid leukaemia
		CNS	Central nervous system
Ag	Antigen	**CP**	Coproporphyrin
AHG	Antibody against human globulin	**CPB**	Competitive protein binding
		CPK	Creatine phosphokinase
AIHA	Autoimmune haemolytic anaemia	**Cr**	Creatinine
		CRP	C-reactive protein
ALA	Delta-aminolaevulinic acid	**CSF**	Cerebrospinal fluid
ALL	Acute lymphoblastic leukaemia	**CT**	Computerized tomography
		CWR	Cardiolipin Wasserman reaction
ALT	Alanine aminotransferase	**CXR**	Chest X-ray
AMA	Antimitochondrial antibody		
AML	Acute myeloblastic leukaemia	**DI**	Diabetes insipidus
		DIC	Disseminated intravascular coagulation
A-mode	Amplitude modulation		
AMP	Adenosine monophosphate	**DM**	Diabetes mellitus
ANA	Antinuclear antibody	**DMSA**	Dimercaptosuccinic acid
ANF	Antinuclear factor	**DNA**	Deoxyribonucleic acid
APTT	Activated partial thrombo-plastin time	**DTPA**	Diethylenetriamine penta acetic acid
ASO	Antistreptolysin O		
AST	Aspartate aminotransferase	**ECF**	Extracellular fluid
ATN	Acute tubular necrosis	**ECG**	Electrocardiogram
AV	Atrioventricular	**EEG**	Electroencephalogram
AVF	Augmented voltage foot lead	**ELISA**	Enzyme-linked immunosor-bent assay
AVL	Augmented voltage left-arm lead		
		EMG	Electromyography
AVR	Augmented voltage right-arm lead	**ENA**	Extractable nuclear antigen
		ERCP	Endoscopic retrograde cholangiopancreatography
BAO	Basal acid output	**ESR**	Erythrocyte sedimentation rate
B-mode	Brightness modulation		
CAH	Chronic active hepatitis, congenital adrenal hyper-plasia	**FDP**	Fibrin degradation products
CBG	Cortisol binding globulin	**FEV**	Forced expiratory volume

FSH	Follicle stimulating hormone
FT3	Free triiodothyronine
FT4	Free thyroxine
FTA	Fluorescent treponemal antibody
FTI	Free thyroxine index
FVC	Forced vital capacity
GFR	Glomerular filtration rate
GGT, γGT	Gamma-glutamyltransferase
GH	Growth hormone
GHg	Glycosylated haemoglobin
GPCA	Gastric parietal cell antibodies
G-6-PD	Glucose-6-phosphate dehydrogenase
GTT	Glucose tolerance test
HAI	Haemagglutination inhibition
Hb	Haemoglobin
HB	Hepatitis B
HB$_s$Ag	Hepatitis B surface antigen
HDL	High density lipoprotein
5-HIAA	5-hydroxyindole-acetic acid
HLA	Human leucocyte antigens
HVA	Homovanillic acid
Ig	Immunoglobulin
ITT	Insulin tolerance test
IU	International unit
IVC	Intravenous cholangiogram
IVU	Intravenous urogram
LAP	Leucocyte alkaline phosphatase
LBBB	Left bundle branch block
LDH	Lactate dehydrogenase
LDL	Low-density lipoprotein
LE	Lupus erythematosus
LH	Luteinizing hormone
LH/FSH-RH	Gonadotrophin releasing hormone
MCH	Mean cell haemoglobin
MCHC	Mean cell haemoglobin concentration
MCV	Mean cell volume
M-mode	Motion scanning
MSU	Midstream urine

5′-NT	5′-nucleotidase
OC	Oral cholecystography
OGTT	Oral glucose tolerance test
17-OS	17-oxosteroids
OT	Old tuberculin
PA	Posteroanterior
PABA	Para-aminobenzoic acid
PAO	Peak acid output
PAS	Para-aminosalicylic acid
PBC	Primary biliary cirrhosis
PBG	Porphobilinogen
PCV	Packed cell volume
PEFR	Peak expiratory flow rate
PFT	Pulmonary function tests
pH	Negative logarithm of the hydrogen ion concentration
pK	Negative logarithm of the ionization constant K
PNH	Paroxysmal nocturnal haemoglobinuria
PP	Protoporphyrin
PPD	Purified protein derivative
PRV	Polycythaemia rubra vera
PT	Prothrombin time
PTH	Parathyroid hormone
RA	Rheumatoid arthritis
RAIU	Radioactive iodine uptake
RBBB	Right bundle branch block
RBC	Red blood cell
RCC	Red cell count
RF	Rheumatoid factor
RIA	Radioimmunoassay
RNA	Ribonucleic acid
RPR	Rapid plasma reagin
RV	Residual volume
SAP	Serum alkaline phosphatase
SBE	Subacute bacterial endocarditis
SCAT	Sheep-cell agglutination test
SIADHS	Syndrome of inappropriate antidiuretic hormone secretion
SLE	Systemic lupus erythematosus
SMA	Smooth muscle antibody
SVT	Supraventricular tachycardia

T3	Triiodothyronine
T4	Thyroxine
TBG	Thyroxine binding globulin
TBM	Tuberculous meningitis
TCT	Thrombin clotting time
TIBC	Total iron-binding capacity
TLC	Total lung capacity
TLCO	Transfer factor of lung for carbon monoxide
TPHA	*Treponema pallidum* haemagglutination
TRH	Thyrotrophin releasing hormone
TS	Tropical sprue
TSH	Thyroid stimulating hormone, thyrotrophin
TT3	Total triiodothyronine
TT4	Total thyroxine

TU	Tuberculin unit
T3U	Triiodothyronine uptake
UP	Uroporphyrin
VC	Vital capacity
VDRL	Venereal Disease Research Laboratory
VLDL	Very low-density lipoprotein
VMA	Vanillylmandelic acid
VT	Ventricular tachycardia
WBC	White blood cell, white blood count
WD	Wilson's disease
W-P-W	Wolff–Parkinson–White (syndrome)

Chapter One

PRINCIPLES OF DIAGNOSIS

Doctors will always seek to ascribe abnormal symptoms, physical signs and investigation results to definite disease syndromes. Successful labelling is mainly useful because it indicates the likely prognosis and the treatment which has the best chance of success. It can also fulfil a psychological need in both doctors and patients. This necessary approach can be misleading for many reasons. Biological variability ensures that features typical of one condition are sometimes an unusual manifestation of another. Apparently identical disease syndromes may result from more than one pathology or aetiology. Some signs and tests, such as hypertension and hypercholesterolaemia, indicate risk factors rather than actual diseases. Despite these reservations the need remains to make diagnoses by four main methods: history, examination, investigation and therapeutic trial. They are usually undertaken in that order, but a finding by one method leads to more intensive study by another.

History
This will always be the major diagnostic method. It deals with the disease as seen by the patient. A symptom described can be a more reliable guide to diagnosis than a figure on a piece of paper.

Examination
This costs only time, can be repeated, and is almost entirely safe. It must be systematic. Physical signs are usually missed because they are not sought.

Therapeutic Trial
Every treatment given is a therapeutic trial, as recovery tends to be taken as evidence that the diagnosis was correct and failure to recover prompts reconsideration of the diagnosis. Therapeutic trials are in general insensitive and non-specific diagnostic tools, with

1

some important exceptions such as corticosteroid drugs in polymyalgia rheumatica. The use of drugs may also obscure the clinical picture, making diagnosis more difficult.

INVESTIGATION

There is much that the practising clinician cannot know about the limitations of individual tests and awareness of this ignorance reduces the chance of error. Pathological and radiological investigations are executed by skilled personnel using complex techniques. Human and technical errors are inevitable, as in all branches of medicine. Intra-observer error, in which one person obtains different results on separate occasions from, for example, the same plasma sample is always possible despite careful quality control. Interobserver variation is especially common in radiology. The practicability of a test varies with the time, expense and skill involved in its performance. The accuracy of a test is the nearness with which the result approaches the true result. The precision is the reproducibility of the result on the same sample. In analytical terms, specificity depends on whether only the substance under investigation is measured and sensitivity relates to the lowest result which can be reliably differentiated from zero; however, they have different meanings in the statistical sense, as defined below. On these matters most clinicians will find guidance from laboratory staff helpful.

A close liaison with pathologists and radiologists with regard to the planning and interpretation of an investigation will increase its efficiency. Some important principles are briefly discussed to help the clinician with this communication.

The Reason for the Test

Safe, inexpensive tests such as routine biochemistry and haematology may be used for screening purposes. They may detect conditions such as moderate anaemia or azotaemia which may not even be suspected clinically. Thought becomes necessary when the result has to be interpreted. However, careful thought is required before requesting an expensive or invasive test. One must know which abnormalities are sought, why they might be present, and what one will do if they are present. This knowledge should be communicated to the person carrying out the test.

Common Errors

A result may be erroneous for a variety of reasons. Errors of labelling and identification will always occur and put at least two patients at risk. They may happen at any of the several steps between taking the sample and interpreting the report. Samples must be put into correct prelabelled bottles and taken promptly to the laboratory.

Samples are often taken by incorrect techniques. Blood is occasionally taken from an arm into which an infusion is running. Prolonged venous occlusion before venesection raises the concentration of proteins, cells and protein-bound constituents in the blood. Clenching the fist raises the concentration of pyruvate, lactate and creatine kinase. Phosphate, glucose and some hormone levels vary with the time of day. If blood samples are left standing, potassium, phosphate and lactate dehydrogenase leak from red cells into the serum. Haemolysis has a similar effect. Posture affects the concentration of serum proteins.

Saliva is often sent to the laboratory instead of sputum. Urine collections are notoriously inaccurate, partly because of difficulties with bladder emptying and partly because of the difficulties patients experience in complying with instructions. It must be clearly explained that the first urine is discarded in a timed collection but all other specimens including the last must be included.

Drugs are a major source of difficulty and many patients are taking some prescribed by their doctor and others obtained from the chemist which they may not even consider to be drugs. These drugs may affect both organ function and the analytical method used by the laboratory.

Interpretation of Tests

There can be few tests which when positive indicate the presence of a disease and when negative indicate its certain absence. The discriminatory ability of tests is described in terms of sensitivity, specificity and predictive value.

Sensitivity

This indicates the percentage of people who actually have the disease in whom a particular test is positive. Ninety-five per cent sensitivity implies 5% false negatives. Increase in sensitivity may reduce specificity. Screening tests should be sensitive.

Specificity

This is the percentage of people without the disease who have a negative test. Ninety-five per cent specificity implies 5% false positives. Specificity is sometimes increased at the cost of sensitivity. Definitive tests should be specific.

Predictive value

The positive predictive value of a test is the percentage of positive results that are true positives and indicate the presence of the suspected disease. It depends not only on the specificity of the test but also on its sensitivity and especially on the prevalence of the disease in the population tested.

If a test has a 90% sensitivity, a 95% specificity and the condition it detects has a 2% prevalence in a given population, the following statements apply. Of 1000 subjects 20 have the disease, 18 will be detected and there will be 5% of 980 or 49 unaffected subjects with false positive tests. Thus there will be a total of 67 positive tests, only 27% of which are true positives. If the prevalence of that disease is 20% in another population, then 200 subjects have the disease and, using the same test, 180 are detected, there are 40 false positives and 82% of all positive results are true positives. It follows that careful selection of patients for study will increase the usefulness of a positive test. Patients with rheumatoid factor in the blood are more likely to have rheumatoid disease if they have polyarthritis and morning stiffness than if they have headache. It does indicate that abnormal results obtained by screening tests must be treated with circumspection. Similar considerations apply to the negative predictive value, the percentage of negative tests that are true negatives.

Range of Normal

The range of normal given for laboratory tests usually includes 95% (two standard deviations from the mean) of a healthy adult (European) population. Therefore only one in forty will be higher and one in forty lower, so a slightly abnormal result may be normal for that patient but not a markedly abnormal result. Also, a result near the edge of normal may be abnormal for that individual. Narrowing of the normal range may be possible if the population group is more clearly defined with regard to sex, age, race and pregnancy. Serum urea levels are higher in the old and lower in pregnancy. With some tests, methods differ between laboratories and the local normal results will vary.

Slightly Abnormal Results

The slightly abnormal result requires careful assessment.

1. The test should be repeated. First, technical error is possible. Secondly, even if the test is reproducible to within 5%, this means that the scatter of results which always occurs must occasionally throw up one still further from the true value.
2. Examination of previous results may indicate a change or trend to be confirmed by further results.
3. The result may be highly relevant and give partial confirmation of a strongly suspected diagnosis or it may be completely irrelevant to the clinical situation. A third possibility is that it suggests some pathology not previously suspected. An example of these three situations might be the finding of a slightly raised aspartate transaminase concentration in a patient with chest pain, in a healthy person, or in a secret drinker.
4. Alternative tests may confirm or refute the suggested information. Reticulocytosis may confirm that a slightly raised bilirubin is related to haemolysis.

BIOCHEMICAL METHODS

Analysis by measurement of weight, volume and titration has been increasingly superseded by the tests below, which in general require less time and skill or are more readily automated. Analysis may involve separation of the component of interest, followed by a method of measuring the substance and then determining the endpoint. Some major methods in use are outlined below.

Colorimetry

The absorption of monochromatic light by a coloured solution is measured photoelectrically.

Spectrophotometry

White or ultraviolet light is split into its component wavelengths, a narrow spectrum is selected and the absorbance of this band by the test substance is measured photoelectrically.

Flame Photometry

A substance is sprayed into a flame which then emits light of a characteristic wavelength. Its intensity is measured photoelectrically. Sodium, potassium and lithium can be measured by this method.

Alternatively, the absorption of energy of specific wavelengths by heated atoms can be determined and this method can be used for calcium, magnesium, copper and iron.

Fluorimetry

When ultraviolet light strikes certain substances in solution they themselves emit light or fluoresce. This is a very sensitive technique useful for steroids and catecholamines, but many drugs cause a non-specific interfering fluorescence.

Nephelometry

The measurement of light scattering by particles in suspension is used in the study of blood lipids and immunological reactions.

Electrometry

Electrodes are used for the measurement of blood gas tensions and hydrogen ion concentration. Changes in proton or electron concentration induce an electric current measured by a sensitive electrometer.

Chromatography

The test serum or extract is applied to a separating medium. Passage of a liquid or gas now separates the components of interest by reason of their solubility, molecular size, or ion exchange affinity. The resolved components are identified in various ways.

Electrophoresis

Charged molecules held on a supporting medium such as paper move at different rates through a liquid phase under the influence of an applied electric field. The separated components are identified by dyes or other means. The technique is applied particularly to proteins.

SEROLOGY AND IMMUNOLOGY

Immunological methods are used in the investigation of many types of disease. Antibodies arise as a result of infection, contact with other foreign material such as drugs, or spontaneously against the cells or organs of the body. Hormones and other proteins can act as immunogens and can be measured by tests involving combination with specific antibodies. The titre of an antibody is expressed as the highest dilution of the serum which gives a positive reaction.

Agglutination
Cells clump and deposit on exposure to an antibody which reacts with a surface antigen. Soluble antigens can be recognized by coating red cells or latex particles with them before exposure to antibody.

Precipitation
Dissolved antigen and antibody form a visible precipitate when mixed in optimal proportions.

Complement-fixing Antibodies
An antigen–antibody reaction may fix complement. It is possible to detect that complement fixation has occurred, and therefore that complement fixing antibodies are present, by using an indicator system. This is a different antigen and antibody which will form a recognizable combination only if complement is still available.

Radial Immunodiffusion (Mancini)
Antigen diffuses out of a well cut in an agar plate which has specific antibody incorporated. The distance of the line of precipitation from the well depends on the amount of antigen in the well. This can be used for immunoglobins (Ig) and complement components.

Double Diffusion (Ouchterlony)
Antigen and antiserum diffuse out from different wells. The further the line of precipitation is from the antigen well, the greater is the concentration of antigen.

Immunoelectrophoresis
In one-dimensional electrophoresis, the sample migrates under the influence of the electric field into a gel of monospecific antiserum and the height of the precipitation arc is related to concentration.

In two-dimensional electrophoresis, the components are electrophoresed first in one direction and then at right angles into agar containing antiserum active against two or more of the components under study, so that two or more arcs form if they are present. Concentration of the test substances is proportional to the area under the arcs. This technique is used in some complement studies.

Immunofluorescence

Antigen fixed to a solid phase combines with antibody in test serum. The antibody is then reacted with fluorescein-labelled IgG and examined under ultraviolet light. Organ-specific antibodies and non-organ-specific antibodies, such as antinuclear factor, can be measured. Biopsy material may be directly examined by labelled anti-Ig to locate Ig fixed to the tissue.

Competitive Protein Binding (CPB)

Test serum containing an unknown quantity of the antigen is incubated with a known amount of the same antigen with an enzyme or radioactive label and a known amount of specific antibody or resin. The binding of labelled antigen is inversely proportional to the amount of unlabelled antigen in the test serum.

Radioimmunoassay (RIA)

Reactions between an antigen and an antibody can be sensitively detected if a radioactive isotope is linked to either. Therefore, trace amounts of either in test serum can be accurately measured. Usually the antigen is labelled and reacted with serum antibody. Labelled free antigen is separated from the labelled antigen–antibody complex by physical or chemical methods. The partitioning of the activity indicates the concentration of antibody in the test solution. This technique is widely used in hormone assays.

Enzyme-linked Immunosorbent Assay (ELISA)

An enzyme whose action is easily measured is coupled to a specific antibody and therefore acts as a marker for the antigen against which the antibody is directed. Either a competitive binding technique is used or human antibodies are detected by incubating them with an insoluble antigen and measuring the human globulin bound by reacting it with enzyme-labelled specific anti-human globulin.

IMAGING TECHNIQUES

Conventional radiology is being rapidly supplemented by increasingly sophisticated non-invasive techniques. The approach to a particular problem may depend on local circumstances. Some of the available methods are discussed.

Isotope Studies

These indicate function rather than structure and are complementary to other techniques. For example, bone scans may detect metastases or osteomyelitis before radiological change appears, whereas a treated metastasis might give a normal bone scan because it is inactive while evidence of radiological change remains.

Scans are useful in the study of the liver, spleen, bones, thyroid, kidneys and brain. They are helpful with pulmonary embolism and myocardial ischaemia. Different carrier chemicals are labelled by different isotopes depending on the tissue studied. Gallium is useful in the detection of neoplasms and abscesses.

Ultrasonography

High-frequency sound waves (above the threshold of human hearing) are generated by passing electricity through a piezoelectric crystal. The waves pass into the body and are reflected at interfaces where tissues of different acoustic impedance are met. The returning echoes are detected by the same crystal and generate a recordable electric potential. The greater the difference in acoustic impedance at the interface of the tissues, the more sound is reflected. The distance of the reflecting structures from the beam source is measured by the time taken for the echoes to return.

In A-mode (amplitude modulation) ultrasound, the returning echo shows as a baseline deflection. This is used to detect the position of midline structures in echoencephalography. In B-mode (brightness modulation) scanning, the echo shows as a dot, the brightness of which is proportional to the intensity of the echo. A plane of reflecting surfaces is imaged, with a moving probe providing a cross-section of structure.

In M-mode (time–motion) scanning, the movement of the dots is watched over a period of time. This is used in echocardiography. Grey-scale imaging shows interfaces within an organ as shades of grey on the screen, revealing internal structure. Real-time scanning uses a larger beam than the B-mode to give a fluoroscopic image of a plane of tissues in motion. A rapid signal emission is necessary for this.

The technique is non-invasive. Transverse scans are depicted as if looking from below and longitudinal scans show the cephalic end to the left. Structures are outlined by reflection, not transmission, of waves and mistakes occur when one structure mimics or obscures another. Apart from cardiac studies, the major use is in the abdomen. Areas furthest from air-containing structures are shown best. These include the aorta, kidneys and other retroperitoneal structures. The liver, spleen, diaphragm, biliary tract, pelvis, fetus and placenta are usually well shown. Cysts are well detected and distinguished from solid structures. The technique is still useful in emaciated patients, in whom computerized tomography may be less accurate.

Computerized Tomography (CT)
Computer processing of X-rays demonstrates minor differences of absorption by different tissues and a grey-scale image of a transverse section of the body is produced. Anatomical definition is more precise than with ultrasonography. The technique has many uses, e.g. in neurology and examination of the abdominal viscera. Multiple lesions can be demonstrated and can be better defined than by other techniques. In the abdomen it is less satisfactory with cachectic patients. It is an expensive technique.

Chapter Two

PLASMA PROTEINS AND ENZYMES

PLASMA PROTEINS

Most proteins are synthesized in the liver, but antibodies are produced by lymphocytes and plasma cells.

Serum Total Proteins

Normal
Adults   (ambulant) 64–83 g/l; (recumbent) 60–78 g/l
Neonates   46–74 g/l
Children   62–80 g/l
Pregnancy   a fall of 10 g/l to a plateau at 20 weeks.

Increase
1. Artefactual — stasis in venepuncture arm.
2. Fluid depletion.
3. Hyperglobulinaemia — a paraprotein or a polyclonal rise in γ-globulin (p. 14).

Decrease
This is usually associated with a fall in the serum albumin concentration.

Serum Albumin

Normal

Adults	35–50 g/l
Neonates	30–45 g/l
Elderly	37–47 g/l
Pregnancy	levels fall rapidly in the first trimester and then slowly until term, by a total of about 10 g/l.

Values vary with the method of estimation used.

Increase
1. Artefactual — venepuncture stasis.
2. Fluid depletion.

Decrease
1. Artefactual — blood taken from an arm, with a drip running. Some methods of estimation are affected by jaundice or drugs.
2. Reduced synthesis — severe dietary deficiency, malabsorption, liver disease. Any illness may cause a fall by up to 10 g/l.
3. Increased loss — proteinuria, burns and exudates, protein losing enteropathy.
4. Pre-eclampsia — levels fall by 5 g/l below normal pregnancy level.

Effect of Hypoalbuminaemia

Albumin provides most of the plasma colloid osmotic pressure and a decrease lowers the blood volume, leading to secondary aldosteronism and oedema. Oedema is usual at levels below 20 g/l, but a level over 30 g/l is not usually the sole cause of oedema. Hypocalcaemia occurs but ionized calcium concentration is unaffected (p. 50). Salicylates, penicillin, sulphonamides and warfarin are largely albumin-bound and this bound fraction is inactive. Hypoalbuminaemia may increase the active free fractions.

Serum Total Globulin

Normal

Adults	21–37 g/l
Neonates	slightly lower.

Total globulin concentration can be derived by subtracting albumin from the total protein level. The various globulin components are measured by electrophoresis. Using this method serum proteins are separated into five groups and quantitated, usually approximately; paraproteins may also be detected (Fig. 2.1). Serum is used, as fibrinogen causes a confusing peak.

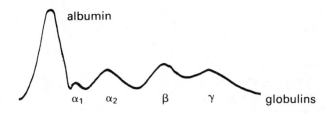

Figure 2.1 The densitometric scan obtained after the electrophoresis of normal serum on cellulose acetate.

Alpha$_1$- (α_1-) Globulin

Normal

Adults	2–3 g/l
Elderly	2–5 g/l
Pregnancy	slightly higher than normal adult.

There is a rise with any tissue damage or inflammation and with oestrogen treatment. A decrease may occur in nephrotic syndrome and with α_1-antitrypsin deficiency.

Alpha$_2$- (α_2-) Globulin

Normal

Adults	4–10 g/l
Neonates	3– 5 g/l
Infants	5– 8 g/l
Elderly	5–12 g/l
Pregnancy	5–12 g/l

An increase is seen in acute stress, nephrotic syndrome, diabetes, hyperthyroidism and adrenal insufficiency. A decrease may occur when albumin synthesis is reduced.

Beta- (β-) Globulin

Normal

Adults	6–10 g/l
Neonates	2– 6 g/l
Infants	5– 8 g/l
Elderly	5–12 g/l
Pregnancy	9–12 g/l

An increase may occur in biliary obstruction and nephrotic syndrome.

Gamma- (γ-) Globulin

Normal

Adults	6–14 g/l
Neonates	adult levels at birth owing to transfer from mother, falling to lower levels in infancy
Elderly	6–16 g/l

All γ-globulins are immunoglobulins (Ig). An increase in Ig production may be polyclonal, demonstrated as a diffuse band on electrophoresis or monoclonal, showing as a narrow band or paraprotein (p. 17).

Increase
A. Polyclonal.
1. Chronic infection.
2. Rheumatoid arthritis (p. 143)
3. Systemic lupus erythematosus.
4. Liver disease (p. 165)
5. Sarcoidosis.

B. Monoclonal (p. 15).

Decrease
1. Protein loss — proteinuria, burns, exudates, enteropathy.
2. Malabsorption.
3. Malnutrition.

4. Haematological malignancy — normal Ig production may be suppressed, but a monoclonal peak may be present.
5. Congenital hypogammaglobulinaemia.

Immunoglobulins (Ig)

These high molecular weight proteins are produced by the plasma cells and lymphocytes as part of the immune response against foreign material such as infecting organisms. Usually several cell types proliferate and there is a polyclonal response producing heterogenous Ig. With neoplasms of these cells a monoclonal proliferation occurs. Ig of a single type is produced and is detected as a paraprotein (p. 17), but levels of normal Ig may be reduced. Five types of Ig are produced and most are γ-globulins. Deficiency of IgG, IgA and IgM can be associated with infection. Measurement is by radial immunodiffusion, though IgD and IgE are present in small quantity and are best measured by radioimmunossay. Serum samples are used.

IgG

Normal
Adults   7–15 g/l; higher in Blacks.
Neonates   adult levels initially, except in prematurity.
Infants   3–12 g/l.

IgG forms about 75% of total Ig. An increase is seen with infections, autoimmune conditions such as SLE and Hashimoto's disease and liver disease (p. 165). Low levels occur in the nephrotic syndrome and congenital deficiency. Normal IgG may be reduced in haematological malignancy, although a paraprotein may be present. Qualitative IgG defects can be detected by failure of response to immunization and the absence of certain natural antibodies, e.g. antibodies to *E. coli.*

IgA

Normal
Adults   1.5–2.5 g/l
Neonates   0   –0.02 g/l

| Infants | 0.1–1.1 g/l |
| Children | 0.2–2.0 g/l |

An increase is seen in portal cirrhosis, especially alcoholic, chronic infections, IgA nephropathy and autoimmune disorders. Gammopathies may cause a monoclonal increase. A decrease is seen in hereditary deficiency, protein-losing conditions or is induced by gold, phenytoin or penicillamine treatment.

IgM

Normal

Adults	0.4–1.8 g/l
Neonates	0 –0.3 g/l
Infants	0.1–1.5 g/l
Children	0.3–1.3 g/l

The first antibody response to antigen is IgM and the presence of antibodies of this class suggests acute infection or re-infection, whereas IgG antibodies may be related to previous infection. Levels are high in chronic infection, biliary cirrhosis and connective tissue disorders, e.g. rheumatoid arthritis. A monoclonal increase is typical of macroglobulinaemia. Reduced levels occur with protein loss.

IgE

Normal
100–200 μg/l

The detection of high levels is most useful in the demonstration of an atopic diathesis (p. 210).

Increase
1. Extrinsic asthma.
2. Allergic rhinitis.
3. Parasitic infestation.
4. Atopic dermatitis.
5. Miscellaneous — cirrhosis, coeliac disease, paraproteinaemia, glomerulonephritis.

IgD

Normal
0–150 mg/l

Some myelomas produce an excess of IgD.

Paraproteins

A homogeneous band of one Ig class is discovered on electrophoresis, usually in the γ-globulin region and usually IgG, IgM or IgA. Its presence implies proliferation of a single clone of cells.

Causes

1. Haematological malignancy — usually myelomatosis, but also macroglobulinaemia and rarer types.

   Myelomatosis is a plasma-cell neoplasm usually presenting with bone pain, anaemia and a high ESR. Abnormal amounts of a single type of Ig are produced, usually recognized in the blood as a paraprotein and sometimes in the urine as Bence Jones protein. The bone marrow contains abnormal plasma cells. Hypercalcaemia and renal failure are common.

2. Cryoglobulinaemia.

3. Essential benign paraproteinaemia — about 20% of patients with paraproteinaemia. In these patients the paraprotein level is stable and is below 20 g/l if IgG or below 10 g/l if of another class. The normal immunoglobulins are not reduced and there is no Bence Jones proteinuria.

Bence Jones Protein

This is a low molecular weight protein, usually a paraprotein fragment consisting of the light chains of the Ig molecule. Because of its small size it normally passes through the glomerulus into the urine and is detectable in the serum only in renal failure. It precipitates when urine is heated to 60°C and redissolves on further heating. It is missed by dipstick tests. It is now usually detected by electrophoresis of the urine after concentration. It occurs with myeloma (50% of patients), macroglobulinaemia and other neoplasms.

Macroglobulins

These are globulins with a molecular weight over 400 000. They are usually IgM but may be IgG polymers. They may be detected by the Sia test, in which a drop of serum flocculates when added to boiled distilled water if macroglobulins are present, or by immunoelectrophoresis.

Causes

1. Waldenström's macroglobulinaemia — this is a lymphocyte neoplasm in which large amounts of monoclonal IgM are secreted. There is lymphadenopathy and anaemia. If the large IgM molecules are present in sufficient concentration hyperviscosity of the blood with bleeding, thrombosis, neurological symptoms and peripheral ischaemia occurs.
2. Malignant lymphomas.
3. Collagen diseases.
4. Diseases with high ESR — sarcoidosis, cirrhosis, nephrosis.

Cryoglobulins

These proteins precipitate on being cooled to 4°C and sometimes at higher temperatures. They may therefore be missed unless the blood specimen is taken into a warm syringe and kept at 37°C until the serum has been separated. They may be IgG or IgM, monoclonal or mixed.

Cryoglobulins can occur in lymphoproliferative, autoimmune and infectious disease in association with a high γ-globulin level, an elevated ESR and sometimes a paraprotein. They may cause Raynaud's phenomenon and cutaneous vasculitis if they are present in high concentration or precipitate at temperatures near to 37°C.

Idiopathic mixed cryoglobulinaemia is associated with glomerulonephritis.

Serum Complement

The complement system is a major mechanism by which antigen antibody reaction causes both defensive inflammation and pathological cell damage. It consists of at least nine plasma enzymes activated in sequence (C142356789).

Total haemolytic complement is detected by the lysis of sheep red cells sensitized by rabbit antibody. It is reduced with deficiency of any complement component. Complement components are measured by radial immunodiffusion.

Raised levels of all complement components can occur in any inflammatory condition and are of no significance. Low complement levels occur in certain diseases and may correlate with disease activity. Measurement of complement levels is most useful in the diseases listed below. C3 is present in the largest concentration and its fixation is the key event in the chain. The complement system may be activated at the C3 level by an alternative pathway and in this case C4 levels may be normal and the serum concentration of properdin, a protein in the alternative pathway, is reduced.

Normal
Total complement	75–160 U/ml (plasma)
C3	0.6–1.5 g/l
C4	0.25–0.75 g/l

Serum for these estimations must be separated immediately and stored at −40°C.

Decrease
1. Post streptococcal acute glomerulonephritis — it recovers in six weeks. C4 recovers more quickly.
2. SLE nephritis — decrease is proportional to activity. C3 and C4 are low.
3. SBE nephritis.
4. Membranoproliferative glomerulonephritis — alternative pathway activation.
5. Serum sickness.
6. Liver disease — due to reduced synthesis.

Serum C-reactive Protein (CRP)

Normal
Adults	0–8 mg/l

This is an α-globulin produced during acute tissue destruction and inflammation which precipitates with pneumococcal somatic C-polysaccharide. The test is performed with antiserum against the protein. Lipaemic sera give false-positives. Results roughly parallel the ESR, but become positive more quickly, usually within twenty-four hours of the onset of disease, and become negative more quickly with recovery. The test is not affected by changed physiological states such as pregnancy (unlike the ESR). It is a good monitor of activity in rheumatic fever, rheumatoid arthritis and systemic vasculitis. It may be positive when the ESR is normal in malignancy.

Serum α-fetoprotein

Normal
Adults   < 40 μg/l; undetectable in most assays. Higher
                        in pregnancy.

This is an oncofetal protein, normally synthesized by the fetus but reappearing in the adult in the presence of certain neoplasms. A marked increase (above 500 μg/l) may be found in primary hepatoma, more often in non-Caucasians than Caucasians. A moderate increase (< 500 μg/l) may be found in hepatoma, secondary hepatic carcinoma, tumours of the alimentary tract and gonads, cirrhosis and hepatitis. Levels may be especially high in abnormal pregnancy, e.g. fetal death or neural tube defects.

Serum α₁-antitrypsin

Normal
Adults   23–44 μmol/l

This glycoprotein inhibits proteolytic enzymes. Deficiency is associated with infantile cholestasis, childhood cirrhosis and severe pulmonary emphysema.

ENZYMES

Enzymes are named from the reaction catalysed. They are usually expressed in international units (IU/l, mIU/ml), one unit being the enzyme activity that converts one micromole of substrate per minute under specified conditions. Enzymes are measured in serum or other fluid specimens by a spectrophotometer. Haemolysed specimens are not suitable. Some enzymes have their normal function in the plasma, e.g. the coagulation cascade, but most are released into the plasma following cell damage or activity. Elevation in the serum enzyme levels is not always proportional to the severity of cell damage. Also, the levels reflect present disease activity and do not remain elevated after disease subsides. Most enzymes occur in several tissues and a rise is only diagnostic in conjunction with the full clinical picture. Isoenzymes, proteins catalysing the same reaction but physically different, may define the tissue of origin more clearly. Most enzyme levels are high in the neonate, but the normal adult range is usually reached by three years.

Serum Acid Phosphatase

Normal
Serum separated early and not haemolysed.

Adults   < 8.2 IU/l

This is the only diagnostically specific enzyme and a rise, particularly of the tartrate labile enzyme, which comes only from the prostate, is indicative of a prostatic carcinoma which has extended outside its capsule and is not too anaplastic.

A false-negative may be found if the specimen measured is not freshly drawn. Tartrate lability is worth testing if the elevation is slight.

False-positives
1. Prostatic trauma — elevation for up to a week after rectal examination, catheterization, urinary retention.
2. Alkaline phosphatase — very high, e.g. Paget's disease.
3. Blood disease (tartrate stable moiety rises) — haemolysed specimen, myeloid leukaemia, thrombocythaemia.

Serum Alanine Aminotransferase (ALT, SGPT)

Normal
Adults   2–45 IU/l
Neonates   1.25 × adult

In general, ALT concentrations parallel those of AST (p. 23) but it is less affected by disease of cardiac or skeletal muscle or by trauma. It may rise more than AST with hepatic cirrhosis or hepatic metastases.

Serum Alkaline Phosphatase (SAP)

Normal

Adults	20–90 IU/l
Infants and children	≤ 3 × normal until growth stops.
Elderly	≤ 140 IU/l without discernible cause. (Paget's disease, osteomalacia and metastatic disease should be considered.)
Pregnancy	rise from about 26 weeks to over twice normal.

In adults the enzyme is derived mainly from the liver and in children from bone. The enzyme from bone is heat labile, while that from liver is relatively heat stable. In pregnancy the placenta produces a heat-stable enzyme. 5'-Nucleotidase (5'-NT) measurement can replace tests for heat stability when the source of the enzyme is uncertain. A raised SAP is likely to come from bone rather than liver if it is heat labile and if 5'-NT or gamma-glutamyltransferase (γ-GT) are normal.

Increase
1. Bone disease — the enzyme concentration rises because of increased osteoblastic activity. The highest rises are seen with Paget's disease and bony metastases. Rises also occur in osteomalacia, hyperparathyroidism and primary bone tumours. Osteolytic metastases, as with myelomatosis, and carcinoma of the breast or colon may not cause a rise. A marked rise may be seen in ankylosing spondylitis.
2. Liver disease (p. 163).
3. Pregnancy — the level is higher than usual with twins and in pre-eclampsia.

Decrease
1. Hypophosphatasia.
2. Reduced bone growth — cretinism, vitamin-C deficiency, achondroplasia.

Serum Amylase (p. 155)

Serum Angiotensin-converting Enzyme (ACE)
Blood collected on ice and serum separated immediately.

Normal
5.5–28 IU/l

Raised levels are seen in sarcoidosis, liver disease, silicosis, asbestosis and hyperthyroidism.

Serum Asparate Aminotransferase (AST, SGOT)

Normal
Haemolysed specimens give false high values.

Adults	2–40 IU/l
Neonates	1.5 × adult
Infants	1.25 × adult

The enzyme is more concentrated in cardiac and skeletal muscle than in the liver and is a useful monitor of myocardial damage. It does, however, rise in many other circumstances.

Increase
1. Myocardial damage (p. 173).
2. Muscle damage.
3. Liver disease (p. 164).
4. Drugs — alcohol; several drugs may cause a rise which may be temporary.
5. Haemolysis — if severe.
6. Miscellaneous — trauma, surgery, shock, pre-eclampsia, occult heart failure, hypokalaemia, severe exertion.

Serum Creatine Phosphokinase (CPK)

Normal
Haemolysis must be avoided.

Adults	10–60 IU/l; slightly higher in males and ambulating patients.
Neonates	10–200 IU/l

CPK occurs in high concentration in brain, cardiac and skeletal muscle, and not in lungs, liver, kidney and red blood cells.

Increase
1. Muscle disease — creatine phosphokinase (CPK) is a sensitive

test. Aldolase, lactate dehydrogenase and transaminase concentrations also rise. Particularly high levels are seen in primary muscular dystrophy, myositis and acute myoglobinuria. Lesser rises are seen with myotonia and neurogenic disease, but there is no rise with myasthenia. Elevations occur in several other conditions. In Duchenne-type dystrophy, levels over ten times normal are seen and precede clinical disease, falling considerably in the late stage. CPK levels may be slightly raised in female carriers. Elevations are less marked or absent in the milder types of dystrophy. Increase occurs also after severe exertion, convulsions and intramuscular injections.

2. Myocardial infarction (not pericarditis or pulmonary infarction).
3. Shock.
4. Hypothyroidism.
5. Cerebrovascular accidents.
6. Drugs — slight rises with many drugs, e.g. clofibrate. Marked rises occur with intoxication, especially with alcohol or hypnotics.

Serum Gamma-glutamyltransferase (γ-GT)

Normal

Adult males	0–65 IU/l
Adult females	0–40 IU/l
Neonates	5 × adult

This enzyme occurs in the liver parenchyma and bile-duct epithelium, the pancreas and the kidney. It is a very sensitive test in many circumstances, but this does reduce its specificity.

Increase

1. Liver disease (p. 164).
2. Pancreatic disease — a rise may occur in carcinoma of the head of the pancreas in the absence of jaundice; acute pancreatitis.
3. Drugs — a raised level may indicate enzyme induction. High levels are seen with alcoholism, barbiturates, anticonvulsants, opiates.
4. Myocardial infarction.

Serum Lactate Dehydrogenase (LDH)

Normal
Serum must be separated early and not haemolysed.

Adults	120–300 IU/l
Neonates	2.5 × adult
Infants	≤1.5 × adult
Children	1.25× adult

Like AST and ALT, it is found in many tissues, so that a rise is equally non-specific. It occurs in myocardial infarction, liver damage, blood disease and malignancy. A marked rise (over 1000 IU/l) is seen in:
1. Blood disease — megaloblastic anaemia, haemolysis and leukaemia.
2. Malignant disease — especially widespread metastases.
3. Acute liver congestion.
4. Acute intoxications.
5. Accidental haemorrhage (abruptio placentae).

Lactate Dehydrogenase Isoenzymes
By electrophoresis LDH may be split into five isoenzymes LD_{1-5}. LD_1 (hydroxybutyrate dehydrogenase) comes mainly from cardiac muscle and red cells and is used to test for myocardial infarction.

Chapter Three

ELECTROLYTE DISORDERS

Electrolyte disturbances are common especially in the young and old, in whom they are more dangerous. The symptoms, however, are usually non-specific, so they are often not suspected until reported by the laboratory. Frequently several factors contribute to the severity of a disturbance.

SODIUM

Sodium (Na^+) excretion by the kidneys is controlled by the glomerular filtration rate and aldosterone. There is also a third factor, which may be a natriuretic hormone secreted in response to extracellular fluid (ECF) volume expansion, or which may depend on intrarenal physical changes.

Na^+ is the main ECF cation and changes in the body Na^+ content largely determine the ECF volume. This is because renal water excretion is affected by ECF osmolality more than ECF volume unless the fall in ECF volume is severe. Two consequences follow from this. First, serum Na^+ concentration reflects changes in water balance as much as Na^+ balance. Hypernatraemia more often means water depletion than sodium overload. Hyponatraemia is often a manifestation of salt and water depletion in surgical patients, but in medical patients it is frequently associated with sodium retention, albeit an even greater water retention. Secondly, serum Na^+ concentration is only one factor in assessing the total body Na^+ content, which is related to serum Na^+ concentration × ECF volume. ECF volume is assessed clinically by indirect means.

Serum Sodium

Normal
Adults   136–146 mmol/l

Neonates	134–144 mmol/l
Infants	139–146 mmol/l
Children	138–145 mmol/l
Pregnancy	133–143 mmol/l

Measurement method
Most laboratories use flame photometry or indirect ion-selective electrodes. The number of sodium ions in the total plasma volume is measured. If plasma solids are increased, this gives a concentration considerably lower than the sodium concentration in plasma water, the biologically important value. Plasma solids are increased when lipid, protein or glucose concentrations are high as with diabetes, myeloma, or intravenous nutrition. A normal sodium concentration in plasma water will be recorded as low (pseudohyponatraemia) or a true hypernatraemia may be missed.

A direct-reading, ion-selective electrode, sometimes used in intensive care units, measures the sodium concentration in plasma water usually about 3 mmol higher than the flame-photometer reading, but in the circumstances above it can be considerably higher.

Increase (hypernatraemia)
Hypernatraemia is more likely to occur in old age, infancy or patients with mental impairment, often as a result of several factors leading to water depletion. A typical patient might be elderly, pyrexial, sweating, confused and hyperventilating due to pneumonia.

1. Water depletion — this is the commonest cause and there may also be total body sodium depletion despite hypernatraemia.
   (a) Reduced water intake — seen with coma and confusion in the old and the young.
   (b) Water loss.
      (i) Renal — diabetes insipidus (p.234), hyperosmolar diabetes, hypertonic feeds.
      (ii) Diarrhoea — in infants.
      (iii) Sweating.
      (iv) Hyperventilation.
2. Sodium excess:
   (a) Sodium retention — a slight rise in serum sodium level is seen with primary aldosteronism and sodium-retaining steroids.

(b) Sodium loading — this is iatrogenic. Hypertonic sodium bicarbonate solutions are given for acidosis. Excess protein and sodium may be given in infant milk formulas or tube feeds. The resultant hyperosmolality also causes renal salt and water excretion.

Decrease (hyponatraemia)
1. Sodium depletion — water is lost to maintain osmolality, but when the fall in ECF volume is sufficient, antidiuretic hormone (ADH) is stimulated and hyponatremia results. This occurs after the loss of about 300 mmol of sodium.
   (a) Gastrointestinal — vomiting, diarrhoea, aspiration and fistulae.
   (b) Renal:
      (i) Kidney disease — sodium loss is characteristic of tubulointerstitial rather than glomerular disease, though renal failure of any type may be aggravated by unsuspected sodium depletion. The recovery phase of acute tubular necrosis and obstructive uropathy are situations to watch.
      (ii) Osmotic diuresis — glycosuria.
      (iii) Diuretics — especially in the elderly.
      (iv) Adrenal failure — Addison's disease and occasionally congenital abnormalities of steroid metabolism.
   (c) Skin — in burns both salt and water are lost, whereas in sweating water loss is predominant. Hyponatraemia can occur in either if dextrose is the main replacement fluid.
2. Water loading (overhydration)
   (a) With sodium retention — oedema is present especially in heart and liver disease, but water retention exceeds that of sodium partly due to poor renal perfusion, and partly due to increased antidiuretic hormone secretion.
      (i) Heart failure — hyponatraemia is not unusual in severe heart failure, especially after diuretic therapy.
      (ii) Cirrhosis — if severe.
      (iii) Acute renal failure.
   (b) Without sodium retention — oedema is not obvious as in the absence of excess sodium the water is distributed equally in cells and ECF. The serum urea is normal or low.
      (i) Iatrogenic — intravenous hypotonic fluids, urethral

irrigation. Patients after operation or burns or receiving Pitressin are particularly susceptible.

(ii) Self-induced — beer drinking, compulsive water drinking.

(iii) Inappropriate ADH secretion syndrome (SIADHS). Serum sodium and osmolal concentrations are below normal. The urine is hypertonic and usually contains more than 50 mmol of sodium per 24 h, depending on sodium intake. Serum urate is usually low. Other causes of hyponatraemia, especially ECF depletion, must be excluded. It is seen with neoplasms, in chest disease, especially carcinoma, tuberculosis and abscess, and transiently with any chest infection. It also occurs with intracranial disease and drugs, especially barbiturates, carbamazepine, chlorpropramide, tolbutamide and clofibrate.

3. Endocrine — glucocorticoid and thyroid deficiency.

4. Pseudohyponatraemia (see p. 27).

5. Internal shifts — in hyperglycaemia there is a shift of water out of the cells and in potassium deficiency there is a shift of sodium into the cells. In severe illness sodium may also enter cells (sick cell syndrome). These shifts are difficult to confirm and other causes of hyponatraemia should be considered first.

Effect of changes
Hypernatraemia causes hyperosmolality, which results in cerebral dehydration, leading to confusion and coma. Fatal cerebral haemorrhage may occur and sodium levels of over 160 mmol/l are very dangerous because of this effect on the brain. Thirst occurs but this will not protect infants, confused or unconscious people. The effects of hyponatraemia depend on the speed of onset as well as the severity.

Symptoms are unusual at levels of over 120 mmol/l unless the onset occurs within hours, but below this headache, nausea, confusion, convulsions, cramps and nausea may occur.

Urine Sodium
Excretion depends mainly on Na^+ intake in the absence of visible sweating. In salt depletion, output falls below 10 mmol per 24 h,

provided the loss is not renal in origin. Urine sodium is also low in oedema-forming states, due to secondary aldosteronism.

Evidence of Sodium Depletion

There is usually also chloride and water depletion, indicating isotonic saline as the usual replacement treatment

1. Clinical evidence — there is often a history of vomiting or reduced fluid intake. There is no evidence of circulatory overload. There is relative hypotension, especially postural.
2. Blood tests — hyponatraemia is neither specific nor sensitive, but is still useful evidence of significant depletion. A raised blood urea, especially a raised blood urea:creatinine ratio (p. 231), is suggestive. The haematocrit, haemoglobin and serum protein concentrations rise, often apparent only in retrospect. Serum urate levels tend to be high, whereas they are usually low in SIADHS (p. 29).
3. Urine sodium — this is usually below 10 mmol/l and osmolality is high. The urine Na^+ concentration may be higher if there is renal disease, if an infusion has been started, or if there is obligatory bicarbonate loss due to alkalosis.
4. Therapeutic test — a carefully watched saline infusion reverses the clinical and biochemical features.

Evidence of Sodium Overload

This is usually accompanied by water, so that hypernatraemia is unusual and mainly iatrogenic. It is a clinical diagnosis. Generalized oedema indicates sodium retention whatever the serum sodium level. Other signs include a raised jugular venous pressure, hypertension and evidence of left ventricular failure.

CHLORIDE

As chloride (Cl^-) is to some extent a passive ion maintaining ECF, electroneutrality levels follow the sodium concentration and are inversely proportional to the bicarbonate level. The serum level is necessary for calculation of the anion gap (p. 45).

Serum Chloride

Normal
Adults   95–105 mmol/l
Neonates   93–110 mmol/l

Increase
1. With hypernatraemia — water depletion and hypertonic saline infusion are the main causes. Isotonic saline raises the chloride level.
2. With low bicarbonate levels — hyperchloraemic acidosis (p. 45) and respiratory alkalosis.

Decrease
1. With hyponatraemia.
2. With high bicarbonate levels — metabolic alkalosis and respiratory acidosis.

Effects of decrease
Chloride deficiency does not affect the ECF volume. It does lead to a renal loss of hydrogen ion (p. 42), causing an alkalosis which in turn causes renal potassium loss, so that potassium deficiency is difficult to correct without chloride replacement. It is therefore important that oral potassium supplements are given with chloride not bicarbonate.

POTASSIUM

Potassium (K^+) is largely intracellular and the serum level is an uncertain guide to the body content, being affected as much by movement of the potassium between the ECF and the cells as by the body content itself. For example, diabetic ketoacidosis is associated with simultaneous hyperkalaemia and potassium depletion, so that correction of the acidosis may precipitate hypokalaemia. However, change in the serum potassium level is itself clinically important. The adrenals and kidneys control potassium balance. In the distal renal tubule, sodium is reabsorbed in exchange for K^+ or H^+. Severe hyperkalaemia stimulates aldosterone secretion, which causes increased K^+ loss in the distal tubule. In hypokalaemia, H^+ is lost instead of K^+ and an alkalosis results.

Serum Potassium

Normal
Adults   3.7–5.2 mmol/l
Neonates   3.7–5.0 mmol/l

Infants   4.1–5.3 mmol/l
Children   3.4–4.7 mmol/l

Platelets release potassium when blood clots and the normal K^+ concentration in heparinized plasma is 3.5–4.5 mmol/l. When primary hyperaldosteronism is suspected plasma samples should be examined.

Increase (hyperkalaemia)
Hyperkalaemia may be wrongly diagnosed when the arm is exercised before venesection, the sample is haemolysed or the serum is not separated within two hours. Severe hyperkalaemia is mostly seen in acute renal failure and several causes may operate simultaneously.
1. Reduced excretion
   (a) Acute oliguric renal failure — the rise is especially rapid with excessive tissue catabolism or acidosis.
   (b) Chronic renal failure — usually an iatrogenic problem associated with the use of potassium supplements, salt substitutes containing potassium, and potassium-sparing diuretics. It is seen sometimes when renin release is disturbed (hyporeninaemic hypoaldosteronism) or when the tubules are not responsive to aldosterone.
   (c) Potassium-sparing diuretics — spironolactone, triamterene and amiloride, especially if combined with potassium supplements.
2. Release from cells
   (a) Acidosis — especial danger occurs if respiratory acidosis, e.g. from chest infection or anaesthesia, is added to metabolic acidosis.
   (b) Cell destruction — acute haemolysis, burns, crush injury and tumour lysis.
   (c) Adrenal failure.
3. Potassium administration
   (a) Potassium supplements — with chronic renal failure or if diuresis does not occur in cardiac failure.
   (b) Infusions — large blood transfusions, stored blood and transfusions to infants can cause hyperkalaemia. Potassium added to infusion bottles must be carefully calculated and mixed.

4. Drugs — the potassium-sparing diuretics block excretion. Beta-adrenergic blocking drugs reduce renin release and block muscle potassium uptake. Captopril reduces aldosterone production.

Decrease (hypokalaemia)
1. Potassium depletion
   (a) Poor intake — this aggravates loss from other causes.
   (b) Gastrointestinal loss
      (i) Vomiting — there is some loss due to potassium in gastric juice, but there is mainly increased urinary loss (p. 42).
      (ii) Diarrhoea — colonic fluid is high in potassium. Laxative addiction is an important cause, often missed. A villous adenoma of the colon can cause severe hypokalaemia.
      (iii) Suction and fistulae.
   (c) Urinary loss
      (i) Osmotic diuresis — diabetes mellitus.
      (ii) Tubular diseases (p. 232).
      (iii) Adrenal overactivity — primary hyperaldosteronism and Cushing's syndrome. Secondary hyperaldosteronism (p. 107).
      (iv) Drugs — all diuretics except those known to spare potassium; drugs with activity similar to aldosterone, e.g. synthetic steroids, carbenoxelone and liquorice; carbenicillin and other high-dosage penicillins.
      (v) Metabolic alkalosis — shortage of intracellular H^+ leads to exchange of K^+ instead of H^+ for reabsorbed Na^+ in the distal tubule.
2. Entry of potassium into cells
   (a) Alkalosis.
   (b) Recovery from megaloblastic anaemia.
   (c) Familial periodic paralysis.
   (d) Drugs — insulin, corticosteroids, i.v. salbutamol and other β-adrenergic agonists.

Diagnosis of potassium depletion
If there is no reason for a shift of potassium into the cells, then the degree of depletion is roughly proportional to the serum level. Alkalosis is a clue to mild depletion. ECG changes include T-wave

flattening and a U wave. With extrarenal loss the urinary concentration will be below 20 mmol/l unless there is severe alkalosis. A concentration of over 30 mmol/l suggests primary urinary loss.

Effect of changes
The main danger of hyperkalaemia is ventricular fibrillation. This is preceded by characteristic ECG changes and cardiographic monitoring is useful.

Paraesthesiae, especially around the mouth, and muscular paralysis can occur. Levels of over 6 mmol/l are an indication for treatment and levels of over 7 mmol/l should be lowered rapidly.

In hypokalaemia, cardiac arrhythmias and digitalis toxicity occur. There is lethargy, muscular weakness and ileus, the last being especially important after surgery. A metabolic alkalosis is common and there may be a polyuria due to tubular damage. Obvious symptoms do not usually occur until the K^+ level falls below 2.5 mmol/l.

OSMOLALITY

This is a measure of the number of solute particles in a fluid and unlike specific gravity is independent of their size (p. 233). Antidiuretic hormone controls renal water excretion and therefore serum osmolality.

Osmolality is measured by the reduction in the freezing point or vapour pressure of water caused by fine particles in a solution. As the major factor contributing to serum osmolality is the sodium concentration, a decreased serum osmolality is always associated with hyponatraemia.

Serum Osmolality

Normal
Adults   275–295 mosmol/kg water
Pregnancy   slightly lower

It can be calculated from the formula: serum osmolality (mosmol/kg) = 2 × serum sodium (mmol/l) + serum glucose (mmol/l) + serum urea (mmol/l).

Calculated and measured osmolality
If the measured osmolality is more than 10 mosmol/kg greater than the calculated value, the following possibilities are considered. The serum water content may be decreased, as in hyperlipidaemia and hyperproteinaemia (p. 27). There may be unusual low molecular weight substances in the serum, such as ethanol, methanol, ethylene glycol or mannitol, and the calculation is a useful check for these.

Urine osmolality
The possible extremes are between 50 and 1400 mosmol/kg. A urine osmolality of below 600 with a serum osmolality of over 300 mosmol/kg occurs in diabetes insipidus and tubular damage, whereas a reduced serum osmolality in association with a higher urine concentration suggests SIADHS (p. 29). Osmolality is less than that of serum in most forms of diuresis but equal to it with an osmotic diuresis. Measurements are useful in acute renal failure (p. 238), polyuria (p. 234) and tubular disease.

Chapter Four

ACID–BASE DISORDERS

CHEMISTRY

Acids and Bases
An acid is a hydrogen ion (H^+) donor. A base is an H^+ acceptor. In aqueous solution a strong acid (HA) dissociates completely to H^+ and A^-, its conjugate base. A weak acid, e.g. carbonic acid (H_2CO_3), dissociates much less, yielding fewer H^+.

Buffers
The presence of a buffer in a solution increases the amount of acid or base that must be added to cause a given change in H^+ concentration. A buffer pair consists of a weak acid and its conjugate base and these mop up the H^+ released by strong acids.

$$H^+Cl^- + Na\,HCO_3 \rightleftharpoons H_2CO_3 + NaCl$$
Strong acid + base   Weak acid + neutral salt

pH
The term pH means 'puissance d'hydrogène'. It is the logarithm of the reciprocal of the H^+ concentration, i.e. $\log_{10} 1/[H^+]$ or $-\log_{10}[H^+]$. The pH notation avoids the small numbers involved when $[H^+]$ is expressed in mol/l, a problem more easily solved by expressing $[H^+]$ in nmol/l. Measuring a biological variable by its negative logarithm does not make a difficult subject easier. A small pH change indicates a larger $[H^+]$ in the opposite direction. A pH change of 0.3 is a twofold $[H^+]$ change and a pH change of 1.0 is a tenfold $[H^+]$ change.

pK
The constant K defines the point where a chemical reaction reaches equilibrium. In the reaction $HA \rightleftharpoons H^+ + A^-$ at equilibrium,

$$K\,[HA] = [H^+] \times [A^-]$$

$$K = \frac{[H^+] \times [A^-]}{[HA]}$$

This is the dissociation content of the acid HA. By analogy with pH, the $pK = -\log K$. The stronger the acid, the lower is its pK value.

The Henderson-Hasselbalch Equation

Acid–base disturbances are described mainly in terms of the carbonic acid–bicarbonate (H_2CO_3–HCO_3^-) system. This system is important for three reasons. First, bicarbonate is the major buffer of the plasma. Secondly, it is a good buffer system because its pK is 6.1, near to the usual plasma pH — buffers are most effective when the solution is near to their pK. Thirdly, the carbonic acid concentration depends on the CO_2 tension (PCO_2) which is regulated by the lungs.

$$[H^+] = K_1 \frac{[H_2CO_3]}{[HCO_3^-]}$$

As $[H_2CO_3]$ depends on $[CO_2]$, which depends on PCO_2

$$[H^+] = K_2 \frac{PCO_2}{[HCO_3^-]}$$

In the pH notation

$$pH = pK + \log \frac{[HCO_3^-]}{K_2 \times PCO_2}$$

As the constants are known when two variables are measured, the third can be calculated.

$$pH = 6.1 + \log \frac{[HCO_3^-] \, (mmol/l)}{0.225 \times PCO_2 \, (kPa)}$$

PHYSIOLOGY

Acid Production

Strong acids are produced by cells when sulphate- and phosphate-containing compounds are metabolized. The intermediate products of fat and carbohydrate metabolism are also acids and these accumulate, especially in anaerobic conditions. About 60 mmol per day of H^+ is released and this is excreted by the kidneys. A much larger amount of H^+ is produced by CO_2 release, about 25 000 mmol per day. This CO_2 enters the red cells, where, under the influence of the enzyme carbonic anhydrase, it is rapidly converted to H_2CO_3. The H^+ released is buffered by haemoglobin until it reaches the lungs.

pH

The pH of arterial blood is 7.36–7.44, equivalent to $[H^+]$ of 44–36 nmol/1. One commonly sees clinically pH values between 7.05 and 7.6 and this indicates a $[H^+]$ variation of between 90 and 25 nmol/l. It is clear that $[H^+]$ may fluctuate more than many other blood constituents. Average intracellular pH is probably about 7.0 and usually, but not always (p. 42), parallels extracellular pH.

The pH of the body is protected by the buffer systems, by respiratory regulation of CO_2 excretion, and by renal regulation of H^+ excretion.

The Buffers

The main intracellular buffers are proteins and organic phosphates. In the plasma the main buffer is the carbonic acid–bicarbonate ($H_2CO_3 - HCO_3^-$) system. In the red cells it is haemoglobin, but mainly the $H_2CO_3 - HCO_3^-$ system. In the urine the main buffers are phosphates and ammonia. When a strong acid is buffered the pH is protected, but the situation is not normal because the amount of conjugate base is reduced by conversion to its associated weak acid thus reducing the buffering power of the system. Normality is restored by renal excretion of H^+ and regeneration of HCO_3^-.

The Lungs

When haemoglobin is oxygenated in the lungs it releases H^+. Combining with HCO_3^-, this H^+ forms H_2CO_3, which breaks down to CO_2 and water. The CO_2 produced by metabolism is thereby excreted into the alveoli. Changes in alveolar ventilation alter CO_2 excretion and therefore the alveolar and arterial P_{CO_2} which are in equilibrium. The lungs can therefore change body pH. Ventilation is adjusted by medullary and arterial chemoreceptors.

As large volumes of CO_2 are excreted, acute changes in respiration cause rapid and severe changes in pH. Despite this, changing the

P_{CO_2} cannot fully compensate for a non-respiratory acidosis or alkalosis. The HCO_3^- concentration of the blood is altered and only the kidneys can restore it to normal.

The Kidneys

The renal tubules secrete H^+ into the tubular fluid in exchange for filtered Na^+. The H^+ is derived from H_2CO_3 produced by the hydration of CO_2 catalysed by carbonic anhydrase. This leaves HCO_3^- behind and the net result is equivalent to the reabsorption of the filtered bicarbonate. A high plasma P_{CO_2} accelerates the process and a change in P_{CO_2} produced by respiratory pathology is compensated by the adjustment of renal HCO_3^- excretion.

The tubules can also secrete H^+ into the tubular fluid against a gradient, achieving a minimum pH of about 5. This is important mainly because it allows two major buffers in the urine to function efficiently. Monohydrogen phosphate accepts H^+ and becomes dihydrogen phosphate. Ammonia (NH_3), produced by the hydrolysis of glutamine in the tubules, accepts H^+ to become ammonium ion (NH_4^+), which cannot diffuse back from the tubular fluid. Quantitatively, buffered H^+ excretion is more important than unbuffered H^+ excretion, even in acid urine.

Note that normal H^+ balance is fully restored by the kidneys, which regenerate or excrete bicarbonate and excrete the anions of strong acids.

PATHOPHYSIOLOGY

Disturbances are traditionally discussed in terms of respiratory and metabolic acidosis and alkalosis. This terminology is inexact because changes in renal function are not strictly metabolic changes and P_{CO_2} may be affected not only by respiratory CO_2 excretion but by metabolic CO_2 production (Fig. 4.1).

Respiratory Acidosis

This is caused by CO_2 accumulation due to hypoventilation (p. 206). There is compensatory renal HCO_3^- retention.

Metabolic Acidosis

Addition of H^+ or loss of HCO_3^- causes a fall in $[HCO_3^-]$ and therefore a fall in pH. Hyperventilation causes a compensatory fall in

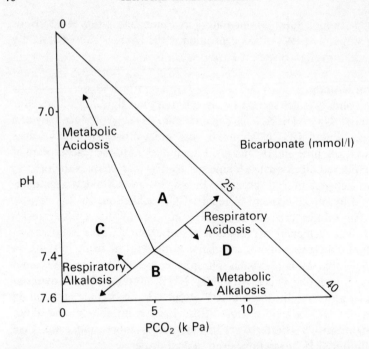

Figure 4.1 Metabolic and respiratory changes. The large arrows show the primary pH and bicarbonate changes and the secondary P_{CO_2} changes in metabolic disturbances and the primary P_{CO_2} and pH changes in respiratory disturbance. The small arrows show the direction of the compensatory bicarbonate and pH changes in respiratory disturbance. Results in areas A and B are always due to mixed respiratory and metabolic disturbance; results in areas C and D might be due to compensated respiratory disturbance.

P_{CO_2} if there is no respiratory problem, but P_{CO_2} does not fall below 2.0 kPa.

Causes

1. Acid gaining — Excessive H^+ production due to metabolic derangement is the usual cause, especially diabetic ketoacidosis, but also lactic acidosis (p. 46), ketoacidosis of starvation and tissue damage, and salicylate intoxication. Also, direct administration of H^+ is seen with ammonium chloride, salicylic acid, and methanol, which last metabolises to formic acid.

Diets high in protein and fat cause increased acid production. Saline infusions dilute plasma bicarbonate.

2. Base losing — all intestinal juices are alkaline and bicarbonate loss is seen with diarrhoea and fistulae. Also, when the ureters are transplanted into the colon or an intestinal loop, chloride is reabsorbed instead of bicarbonate, which is lost.

3. Renal dysfunction — in renal failure of any sort all the mechanisms of renal H^+ excretion tend to be impaired and uraemic anions accumulate. With renal tubular damage there may be a reduced $[H^+]$ gradient between tubular and interstitial fluid.

Aldosterone deficiency reduces H^+ for Na^+ exchange. The carbonic anhydrase inhibitors, such as acetazoleamide, impair bicarbonate reabsorption.

Effects of Acidosis

Severe acidosis depresses cardiac output, promotes arrhythmias and depresses conscious level. Glycolysis is reduced, and potassium comes out of cells, causing hyperkalaemia. A marked leucocytosis may occur. The oxygen dissociation curve of haemoglobin is shifted to the right, improving oxygen delivery to the tissues. Chronic acidosis leaches calcium from bones.

Respiratory Alkalosis

A fall in P_{CO_2} (p. 206) causes a rise in pH and a compensatory fall in plasma bicarbonate owing to reduced renal reabsorption. The compensatory change takes a few days.

Metabolic Alkalosis

There is a rise in HCO_3^-, which causes a rise in pH which may be poorly compensated by hypoventilation.

Causes

1. Soluble base intake — this is seen mainly with sodium bicarbonate infusions but also when bicarbonate is taken orally, especially for indigestion and with lactate or citrate administration.

2. H^+ loss.

   (a) Gastric — vomiting due to pyloric stenosis typically causes a hypochloraemic alkalosis with potassium deficiency. When the pylorus is patent the acid gastric juice is more or less

  mixed with alkaline intestinal juice and alkalosis is less
  marked.
 (b) Renal — excess renal H^+ loss occurs in several circumstances. In the distal tubule K^+ competes with H^+ for
  exchange with reabsorbed Na^+. In potassium depletion H^+ is
  lost preferentially. Also, H^+ enters the cells so an extracellular alkalosis and intracellular acidosis occur.

In chloride (Cl^-) deficiency Na^+ has to be exchanged for H^+
because it cannot be reabsorbed from the tubular fluid along with
Cl^-. There is increased reabsorption of Na^+ in the distal tubule in
exchange for K^+ and H^+, with hyperaldosteronism and administration of corticosteroids or carbenoxelone.

Effects of Alkalosis
It predisposes to K^+ depletion and reduces the ionization of calcium.
Paraesthesiae, tetany and syncope may occur.

MEASUREMENTS

pH

Normal
7.44–7.36

Measurements are usually made on heparinized arterial blood collected with the same precautions as for blood gas analysis (p. 206) and
may be corrected for body temperature. Capillary blood is variably
more acid. The pH meter uses a high conductivity glass electrode
sensitive only to H^+, so it registers a voltage change with H^+ change.

P_{CO_2} (CO$_2$ Tension)

Normal arterial (p. 206)
A rise is seen with ventilatory problems or as a compensatory change
in metabolic alkalosis. A fall is seen with hyperventilation or as a
compensatory change in metabolic acidosis.

Plasma Bicarbonate
There is a rise in metabolic alkalosis, compensated respiratory
acidosis and extracellular fluid depletion. There is a fall in metabolic

acidosis, compensated respiratory alkalosis and ECF dilution. There are three main approaches to measurement and some dispute as to which is best.

1. Total CO_2 (TCO_2)

Normal
22–29 mmol/l in mixed venous blood.
21–28 mmol/l in arterial blood.

Values may be slightly low due to CO_2 loss if blood is stored before measurement. All the CO_2 is driven off by strong acid added to the plasma and this can be measured volumetrically or by titration.

2. Actual Bicarbonate

This is calculated from the Henderson–Hasselbalch (H-H) equation and is fairly close to the TCO_2. It assumes that the H-H constants are valid.

3. Standard Bicarbonate

Normal
21–25 mmol/l

This is the bicarbonate concentration in fully oxygenated whole blood at 37°C equilibrated at a PCO_2 of 5.3 kPa. In practice it is calculated by the Astrup technique.

Standard bicarbonate corrects the actual bicarbonate for changes caused by alteration of the blood CO_2 content. It helps to assess the metabolic component of a combined respiratory and metabolic disorder. In acute respiratory acidosis TCO_2 is slightly raised but standard bicarbonate is normal. In chronic respiratory acidosis TCO_2 is markedly raised. Standard bicarbonate is also raised due to renal bicarbonate retention, but is slightly lower than TCO_2.

Astrup Technique

Astrup and his colleagues devised a method of assessing acid–base balance in arterial blood using in vitro equilibrations and nomograms (Fig. 4.2). The measurements can be carried out on small heparinized samples of arterialized capillary whole blood drawn into capillary tubes. The technique is a little questionable because in vitro manipulations may not truly represent events in the body.

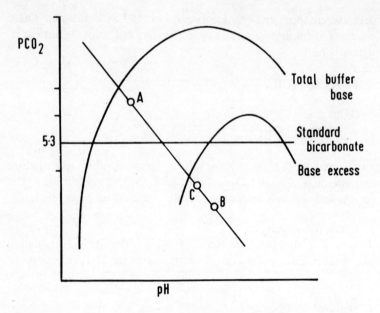

Figure 4.2 Astrup technique. (1) A capillary blood sample is equilibrated at two known $P\text{CO}_2$ concentrations, A and B, and its pH is determined. (2) The line AB is drawn on the $P\text{CO}_2$/pH graph. (3) The pH of the original sample is measured and its $P\text{CO}_2$ is determined from the graph at C. (4) Total buffer base, standard, bicarbonate and base excess are derived from the point where the line AB intersects the calculated lines drawn on the graph.

From it the $P\text{CO}_2$, the standard bicarbonate, the buffer base and the base excess can be calculated.

Buffer base
The normal buffer base can be calculated from the equation:
Normal buffer base = 42 + 0.4 Hb

Hb is expressed in g/100 ml and average values for the normal buffer base lie between 45 and 50 meq/l. It is a measurement of the total buffers available in whole blood, including bicarbonate, protein and haemoglobin. It is measured on the Astrup nomogram as the point at which the log $P\text{CO}_2$–pH line crosses a calculated line drawn on the nomogram (Fig. 4.2).

Base excess

Normal

Adults	$\pm$ 3 mmol/l
Neonates	-10 to -2 mmol/l
Infants	-7 to -1 mmol/l
Children	-4 to $+2$ mmol/l

It is the difference between the observed buffer base and the normal buffer base and may be positive or negative, when it is called a negative base excess or base deficit. It is the point on the Astrup nomogram where the log PCO_2–pH line crosses the base excess line. The base excess line is derived from the effects of adding varying amounts of acid or base to plasma or blood. Changes in it are parallel to but slightly greater than changes in standard bicarbonate and both give an indication of the metabolic component of an acid–base disturbance.

Anion Gap

Normal
11–19 mmol/l

The sum of positive and negative charges in the plasma is equal, but the sum of the main measured cations Na^+ and K^+ is greater than the sum of the measured anions Cl^- and HCO_3^-. This is the anion gap, filled normally by protein, phosphate, sulphate and urate. It is calculated from four different measurements, so an error of 5 mmol/l must be expected.

The anion gap usually rises because serum bicarbonate concentration falls in metabolic acidosis. This is usually due to the presence of uraemic anions or keto-acids, but also occurs in lactic acidosis and with poisons which increase the formation of organic acids (p. 40). Hyperchloraemic acidosis, with a normal anion gap, occurs in renal tubular acidosis, loss of intestinal juices, ureteric transplantation and treatment by carbonic anhydrase inhibitors. Carbenicillin sodium raises the anion gap by depressing chloride levels.

A reduced anion gap may occur in multiple myeloma, where the proteins may act as cations, in hypoalbuminaemia, which increases chloride and bicarbonate concentrations, in bromism, which gives falsely high chloride levels, and in pseudohyponatraemia.

Blood Lactate

Normal
Heparinized whole blood

Arterial   0.5–1.6 mmol/l;   venous 0.5–2.2 mmol/l

Glucose and amino-acids are broken down to pyruvate, which is further metabolized in the tricarboxylic acid cycle. Abnormal metabolism may divert pyruvate into lactate or ketone bodies. Lactic acidosis should be suspected when an ill patient has a metabolic acidosis inappropriate to the degree of uraemia or ketonaemia. There is an unexplained anion gap (p. 45). Usual criteria are a pH below 7.25 and a blood lactate of over 5 mmol/l.

Lactic acidosis is seen in tissue hypoxia, as with all forms of shock, left ventricular failure and severe anaemia. It also occurs in liver failure, renal failure and uncontrolled diabetes, as well as severe infection and leukaemia. The biguanides, especially phenformin, cause it, particularly with older patients, large doses, renal failure and alcohol ingestion. Ethanol ingestion, fructose and other carbohydrates used in parenteral nutrition are other causes.

Urine pH

The urine is not reliably acid in acidosis and alkaline in alkalosis because the pH may change when compensation has been achieved. Also, in hypokalaemic alkalosis the urine may, paradoxically, be acid due to preferential secretion of H^+ by the distal tubule.

CLINICAL ASSESSMENT

Preliminary

Acid–base disturbances usually occur as part of a systemic illness. When they are suspected preliminary assessment involves measurement of the concentration of bicarbonate, other electrolytes, glucose and urea in venous blood, and testing the urine for sugar and ketones. These results added to the total clinical picture will usually define adequately the nature, severity, cause and appropriate treatment of an acid–base disturbance, particularly in uncomplicated metabolic problems, such as renal failure, vomiting or chronic stable respiratory acidosis. In diabetes mellitus plasma pH and ketones should also be measured.

Electrolytes
Further clues may be obtained from perusal of the electrolytes. Acidosis usually causes hyperkalaemia. The combination of hypokalaemia and acidosis may, however, be seen with diarrhoea, renal tubular disease and treatment with carbonic anhydrase inhibitors.

Where a low potassium is seen together with a high bicarbonate the situation is usually one of alkalosis secondary to hypokalaemia, rather than the reverse. A high bicarbonate in respiratory disease is usually an indication of compensated respiratory acidosis. After treatment with diuretics the high bicarbonate may reflect a hypokalaemic alkalosis. Where acidosis is associated with a normal anion gap and usually a high chloride the causes of hyperchloraemic acidosis should be considered. Where the anion gap is widened but there is neither ketoacidosis nor uraemic acidosis sufficient to explain the degree of acidosis, conditions such as lactic acidosis or poisoning (p. 40) must be considered.

Detailed Analysis
This is necessary in any complicated problem, particularly where there is acute respiratory acidosis or a mixed metabolic and respiratory disturbance. Bicarbonate, PO_2, PCO_2 and pH should be measured directly on an arterial blood sample. Fig. 4.1. may be helpful in analysing the disturbance. A starting point is to see whether pH is high or low. A raised bicarbonate would be expected in a respiratory acidosis unless the condition is of less than a day's duration. If it is not raised, there is probably a metabolic acidosis also. The PCO_2 falls in metabolic acidosis unless there is also respiratory disturbance. Where respiratory acidosis is combined with metabolic alkalosis PCO_2 and $[HCO_3^-]$ may be markedly raised, with a low PO_2 and a relatively normal pH. If the results are difficult to interpret they should be rechecked in case there is a laboratory error.

Derived values
By the Astrup technique base excess, standard bicarbonate and buffer base may be used to disentangle acid–base disturbances (p. 43). There is, however, a case for managing patients entirely by the clinical picture and repeated direct measurements.

Treatment

The bicarbonate deficit in a metabolic acidosis may be calculated as follows:

$$\text{Deficit (mmol)} = 0.5 \times \text{body weight (kg)} \times \text{fall in } [HCO_3^-] \text{ (mmol/l)}$$

It is suggested that half the deficit be replaced. In practice this can be unreliable. A lactic acidosis may require large amounts of bicarbonate. If bicarbonate is given in diabetic keto-acidosis, dangerous overcorrection and hypokalaemia may occur. It is always wise to recheck pH and serum potassium two to three hours after treatment has started in a severe acid–base disorder. It is also true that if the general condition of the patient and the function of organs is improved, an acid–base disturbance will begin to correct itself.

Effects of treatment

Changes in $P\text{CO}_2$ follow changes in ventilation rapidly, but the adjustment of the plasma bicarbonate concentration takes a few days. CO_2 crosses cell membranes and the blood-brain barrier readily, but bicarbonate does not. Rapid correction of a chronic respiratory acidosis by artificial ventilation may produce a metabolic alkalosis because of the high bicarbonate concentration. A patient whose $P\text{CO}_2$ is kept at a low level by artificial ventilation will excrete bicarbonate. When taken off the ventilator metabolic acidosis and hyperventilation may occur. When bicarbonate is given in metabolic acidosis it penetrates slowly into the CSF. If the effect on arterial chemoreceptors stops hyperventilation, CSF $P\text{CO}_2$ rises with CSF acidosis and depression of conscious level. Correction of acidosis also shifts the haemoglobin–oxygen dissociation curve to the left, with reduced oxygen delivery to the tissues. Severe acidosis therefore requires rapid partial but a more gradual total correction.

Chapter Five

CALCIUM, PHOSPHATE AND MAGNESIUM DISORDERS

CONTROLLING HORMONES

Vitamin D
Vitamin D promotes calcium and phosphate absorption from the gut and is involved in bone mineralization and bone resorption. Vitamin D is manufactured in the skin under the influence of ultraviolet light and is also absorbed from the duodenum and jejunum. In the liver the provitamin is converted to 25-hydroxy vitamin D. In the kidney this is further converted to 1,25-dihydroxy vitamin D, the active hormone. Parathyroid hormone is necessary for this transformation. Deficiency of active vitamin D causes rickets in children, osteomalacia in adults, and may cause myopathy. An excess causes hypercalcaemia.

Parathyroid Hormone (PTH)
PTH raises the plasma calcium level by mobilizing it from bone and by increasing renal tubular reabsorption. Through its action on vitamin D metabolism calcium absorption from the gut is indirectly promoted. Renal tubular phosphate reabsorption is decreased, so the plasma phosphate concentration falls.

Calcitonin
Calcitonin lowers the serum calcium concentration by inhibiting osteoclastic bone resorption and by a direct calciuric effect on the kidney. It is secreted by the parafollicular cells of the thyroid in response to hypercalcaemia.

BIOCHEMICAL VALUES

Serum Calcium

Normal
Clotted blood taken without prolonged venous stasis.

Adults	2.20–2.60 mmol/l
Neonates	1.90–3.5 mmol/l
Infants	2.50–3.0 mmol/l
Elderly	in females up to 2.75 mmol/l
Pregnancy	a 10% fall due to the fall in serum albumin

Correction factor — subtract or add 0.02 mmol/l for each 1 g/l the serum albumin deviates from 40 g/l or from the midpoint of the normal laboratory range. The serum calcium is about 50% ionized and most of the rest is protein bound.

The ionized moiety is biologically important but not easily measured. It is therefore necessary to correct the total serum calcium level for changes in the protein concentration by the approximate correction factor. It is not valid where serum protein levels are markedly abnormal or where there are acid–base disturbances. Acidosis increases the ionized calcium percentage and alkalosis reduces it. Serum calcium levels represent a balance between calcium absorption and renal excretion and bone resorption and bone mineralization.

Increase (hypercalcaemia)
1. Neoplasms — the commonest cause
   (a) Metastatic bone disease — especially with osteolytic secondary deposits from breast, lung or kidney tumours and multiple myelomatosis. It can occur with lymphomas, rarely with prostatic or thyroid neoplasms. The alkaline phosphatase level (SAP) is high or very high except with myelomatosis, where it is usually normal because there is no osteoblastic response. X-rays or bone scans may be positive.
   (b) Pseudohyperparathyroidism — secretion by the tumour of a hormone with activity similar to PTH typically occurs with squamous cell bronchial carcinoma but also with hypernephroma and other tumours. The SAP may be normal.

There is usually a response to prednisolone (p. 57) or removal of the tumour.

2. Primary hyperparathyroidism (p. 56).
3. Drugs — vitamin D is given in high dose in renal failure and hypoparathyroidism, sometimes unwisely in other conditions and sometimes self-administered. The effect is cumulative and hypercalcaemia may appear after months of apparent stability. Infantile hypercalcaemia due to vitamin D supplementation of bottle feeds is seen less now. Thiazide diuretics, which reduce calcium excretion can cause mild hypercalcaemia, which disappears within a few weeks of stopping the drug. The milk–alkali syndrome is rarely seen now as non-absorbable antacids are used, so the combination of hypercalcaemia and peptic ulcer should suggest a parathyroid adenoma, although large doses of calcium salts may be responsible. Calcium resins in renal failure are a possible cause.
4. Sarcoidosis.
5. Endocrine — acromegaly, severe thyrotoxicosis, Addison's disease.
6. Immobilization — especially in children and Paget's disease.
7. Dehydration.
8. Familial benign hypercalcaemia.

Decrease (hypocalcaemia)
An adjustment must be made for the serum albumin level. Phosphate levels are low in vitamin D deficiency and high in renal failure and hypoparathyroidism.
1. Vitamin D deficiency (p. 49).
2. Renal failure (p. 56).
3. Hypoparathyroidism — this may be seen after partial thyroidectomy or radioactive iodine treatment and after removal of a parathyroid adenoma. In the latter case calcium is deposited in the diseased bones. Idiopathic or autoimmune hypoparathyroidism also occurs. In these conditions the serum phosphate is generally high and the parathyroid hormone (PTH) level is low. In pseudohypoparathyroidism the biochemistry of hypoparathyroidism is associated with high PTH levels, PTH resistance and skeletal abnormalities.
4. Paediatric — in the newborn, due to maternal diabetes, osteomalacia or hyperparathyroidism.

5. Drugs — oestrogens antagonize PTH. Anabolic steroids, carbenoxolone, anticonvulsants (p. 56), oral phosphates and calcitonin can lower calcium levels.

Effect of changes
Hypercalcaemia can cause damage to the renal tubules, leading to polyuria and polydipsia. Renal calculi and renal failure may occur. There may also be anorexia, nausea, vomiting, constipation, headache, personality change and ECG changes. There is long-term danger in sustained levels over about 2.80 mmol/l and immediate danger of cardiac arrest with levels over about 3.75 mmol/l. When hypercalcaemia is associated with hyperphosphataemia there is an increased danger of metastatic calcification.

Hypocalcaemia increases the excitability of peripheral nerves causing numbness and paraesthesiae, especially of the fingers, tetany and even stridor in infants. Depression and irritability occur. PTH secretion is stimulated. Cataracts occur in chronic cases.

Urine Calcium

Normal

Adult males	2.5–7.5 mmol per 24 h.
Adult females	2.5–6.2 mmol per 24 h.
Children	< 0.15 mmol/kg per 24 h.

These values refer to normal diets. Excretion is lower on a calcium-restricted diet.

Increase (hypercalcuria)
1. Hypercalcaemia of any cause.
2. Idiopathic hypercalcuria — usually detected because of stone formation.
3. Renal tubular defects.
4. Immobilization.
5. Sarcoidosis.
6. Drugs — corticosteroids, frusemide.

Decrease
1. Hypocalcaemia.
2. Osteomalacia.

3. Renal disease — nephrotic syndrome, acute nephritis, renal failure.

Serum Phosphate

Normal
Clotted blood taken in the fasting state.

Adults	0.70–1.45 mmol/l
Neonates	1.1 –2.8 mmol/l
Infants	1.4 –2.2 mmol/l
Children	1.4 –1.8 mmol/l

The phosphate level is more variable than that of calcium. False high values are seen if the blood is haemolysed or stands unseparated because of leakage from cells.

Increase (hyperphosphataemia)
1. Renal failure.
2. Diabetic ketosis.
3. Vitamin D excess.
4. Hypoparathyroidism.
5. Healing fractures.
6. Miscellaneous — acromegaly, haemolysis, neoplasms.

Decrease (hypophosphataemia)
1. Vitamin D deficiency.
2. Hyperparathyroidism.
3. Drugs — phosphate enters the cells when dextrose infusions or insulin are given and concentrated carbohydrate solutions may cause severe hypophosphataemia. Aluminium hydroxide, oestrogens, sex hormones and anabolic steroids are other causes.
4. Nutritional deficiency — most diets contain adequate phosphate, but this may not be so with patients on prolonged i.v. infusions or nasogastric suction. Vomiting and alcoholism may cause deficiency.
5. Renal tubular disease (p. 232).
6. Acute infection — especially Gram-negative bacterial septicaemia.

Effects of changes in serum phosphate
Primary hyperphosphataemia causes reciprocal lowering of the serum calcium. In severe hypophosphataemia there may be paraesthesiae, fits, weakness and coma, and this is seen especially with parenteral nutrition. Chronic hypophosphataemia in renal tubular disease may cause rickets.

Urine Phosphate

Normal
29–42 mmol per 24 h.

Phosphate excretion falls when intake is reduced. Normally about 85% of the phosphate filtered by the glomeruli is reabsorbed in the proximal tubules. Reabsorption is reduced and excretion is increased in hyperparathyroidism, acidosis, immobilization and certain renal tubular disorders. Excretion is reduced in hypophosphataemia, hypoparathyroidism, hypervitaminosis D and renal failure. Tubular reabsorption can be calculated by relating the phosphate clearance to the creatinine clearance. Indices relating tubular phosphate reabsorption to the serum phosphate level have been used in the diagnosis of hyperparathyroidism, but they are not reliable.

Serum Magnesium

Normal
Adults   0.70–1.20 mmol/l
Neonates   may be lower.
Pregnancy   about 15% lower.

Magnesium moves into and out of bone with calcium because it occurs in bone mineral, and it moves between cells and ECF with potassium and phosphate, all three being present in higher concentration in the cells than in the ECF.

Increase
This is seen in renal failure with hyperkalaemia especially if magnesium is given as a cathartic or antacid and also in hypercalcaemia.

Decrease
1. Gastrointestinal loss — severe diarrhoea is the commonest cause, but also malabsorption and nasogastric aspiration.
2. Reduced intake — malnutrition, i.v. feeding, alcoholism.
3. Hypocalcaemia — especially after parathyroidectomy.
4. Hypokalaemia — diuretics and primary aldosteronism.
5. Drugs — diuretics, gentamicin, cisplatin.

Effect of changes in serum magnesium
Hypermagnesaemia causes drowsiness, loss of tendon reflexes and cardiac depression. Hypomagnesaemia causes neuromuscular irritability, depression, nausea, ventricular arrhythmias, resistant atrial fibrillation, digitalis toxicity, hypocalcaemia and hypokalaemia. It may be relatively common in older patients taking diuretics.

CLINICAL PROBLEMS

Bone Disease
Clinical diagnosis is made from X-rays and biochemical changes but sometimes, particularly in mild cases, histology is necessary.

Paget's disease
Normal bone is broken down and replaced by vascular primitive bone. The disease is recognized radiologically and affects especially the spine, pelvis, skull and femur. It is rare before the age of forty. The serum alkaline phosphatase is often greatly raised, but hypercalcaemia is very rare and only seen with immobilization.

Osteoporosis
Bone density is reduced per unit volume. The diagnosis is radiological, but subjective and difficult. There are no biochemical changes. Osteoporosis is usually diagnosed when fractures occur.

Hyperparathyroidism
Increased osteoclastic activity predominates and subperiosteal erosions and bone cysts occur. With primary hyperparathyroidism, hypercalcaemia is present. Secondary hyperparathyroidism is caused by a fall in serum calcium concentration. When it is due to osteomalacia, phosphate levels are low, but in renal failure they are high.

Rickets and osteomalacia

The organic bone matrix (osteoid) does not calcify, causing soft bone and wide osteoid seams. In rickets the epiphyseal cartilage fails to calcify. Changes of secondary hyperparathyroidism also occur. Decalcified areas are recognized on X-ray.

The disease is commonly due to vitamin D deficiency caused by poor diet and lack of sunlight. It is also seen with malabsorption. Anticonvulsants affect hepatic, and renal damage affects renal vitamin D activation (p. 49). Renal tubular disease reduces bone mineralization by causing hypophosphataemia. Some of the biochemical changes precede radiological signs but are not entirely reliable. The serum calcium level may be only slightly low and often rises to low normal owing to secondary hyperparathyroidism. The phosphate level tends to be low except in renal failure. Serum alkaline phosphatase is usually high but may be raised for other reasons. Urine calcium excretion below 2.5 mmol per 24 h and especially below 1.2 mmol per 24 h is suggestive in the absence of renal disease. It is rarely necessary to measure the 25-hydroxy-D level, normally about 10–40 ng/l.

Azotaemic osteodystrophy

The biochemical and histological disturbance is complex. Usually either osteomalacia or secondary hyperparathyroidism predominate and metastatic calcification can occur if the calcium phosphate product is high. Severe renal damage impairs activation of vitamin D. Also, a fall in glomerular filtration rate causes a rise in serum phosphate which is deposited with calcium in bone. The fall in serum calcium concentration stimulates PTH secretion which partially restores urinary phosphate excretion and serum phosphate and calcium levels.

Primary Hyperparathyroidism

It usually presents with renal stones or with hypercalcaemia, often found by chance. Both serum ionized calcium and PTH concentrations are high, but reliable measurements of both can be difficult and the diagnosis must often be made by excluding other causes of hypercalcaemia.

1. Serum calcium — hypercalcaemia should be established in several fasting samples taken without stasis and corrected for serum protein changes. A parathyroid adenoma is unlikely in the

absence of hypercalcaema unless there is concurrent vitamin D deficiency or hypercalcaemia has caused renal failure. If these conditions have lowered the serum calcium to normal, the diagnosis is difficult to make. Serum calcium levels fall in winter.

2. Clinical features — longstanding hypercalcaemia without weight loss and with renal stones is suggestive of primary hyperparathyroidism. Occult neoplasms, sarcoidosis and drugs cause particular diagnostic difficulty. These may be suggested by history, examination, weight loss, a high ESR or hyperglobulinaemia.

3. Biochemical features — a high serum phosphate suggests a non-parathyroid cause in the absence of renal failure. Serum chloride is usually slightly high, as high PTH levels produce a mild renal tubular acidosis, whereas they tend to be low when other causes of hypercalcaemia suppress PTH production. A marked rise in serum alkaline phosphatase in the absence of radiological evidence of hyperparathyroidism suggests a neoplastic cause.

Urine calcium excretion is increased in hypercalcaemia, except in renal failure and familial benign hypercalcaemia. The latter condition should be suspected if the serum calcium is between 2.6 and 3.2 mmol/l and urine calcium excretion is below 2.5 mmol per 24 h. A low urinary cyclic AMP excretion rate is evidence against primary hyperparathyroidism.

4. Radiology — the diagnosis may be confirmed in some patients by finding subperiosteal erosions in high quality radiographs of the hands.

5. Corticosteroid suppression test — this test is most useful where the calcium concentration is above 3.0 mmol/l. After three basal calcium estimations prednisolone 20 mg eight-hourly is given orally for ten days, then tailed off. Calcium levels are measured on the last three days, with all values being corrected for changes in the serum albumin concentration. A fall in the calcium concentration to normal is good evidence against primary hyperparathyroidism.

6. Parathyroid hormone (PTH) — a fasting PTH level should be taken for measurement by radioimmunoassay. A high or normal level in the presence of hypercalcaemia suggests primary hyperparathyroidism. Absence of PTH from the plasma casts doubt on the diagnosis. However, the assay available may not be reliable and PTH levels may be slightly high in malignancy.

7. Localization of the tumour — this is usually done by the surgeon at operation, but isotope scans are improving.

Hypercalcaemia and Azotaemia

Typically azotaemia is secondary to hypercalcaemia and responds to treatment of this. Dehydration, especially in the elderly, may cause both mild hypercalcaemia and azotaemia, which will both rapidly respond to fluid replacement. A saline drip will also lower the serum calcium and blood urea when the azotaemia is secondary to hypercalcaemia because of associated fluid depletion, but the calcium level will not return to normal. Control of hypercalcaemia will further lower the blood urea in most instances. However, in chronic cases there may be irreversible renal damage. Rarely tertiary hyperparathyroidism, in which the hypertrophied glands of secondary hyperparathyroidism become autonomous, occurs in chronic renal failure, usually after transplantation or after a fall in the raised phosphate level, and here hypercalcaemia also occurs. Hypercalcaemia can be concurrent with renal damage from other causes.

Chapter Six

VITAMINS AND NUTRITION

Vitamins are organic dietary constituents essential to life but required only in small quantities. Deficiency of the fat soluble vitamins A, D and K occurs in malabsorption. Dietary vitamin deficiency is by no means rare in the United Kingdom and deficiency of vitamins B_1, B_{12}, C, D and folic acid should be considered. Hypervitaminosis D, A and K occur, the first being most common and usually iatrogenic.

Serum Vitamin A

Normal
0.7–1.7 μmol/l

Serum carotene

Adults	1.1–3.7 μmol/l
Infants	0.4–1.3 μmol/l
Children	0.7–2.4 μmol/l

Vitamin A deficiency causes reduced visual dark adaptation, followed by xerophthalmia and keratomalacia. It occurs in malabsorption. Carotene is a vitamin A precursor and its measurement is used as a screening test for malabsorption. A one-month course of vitamin A 50 000 units daily may be used as a therapeutic test for deficiency.

Vitamin B_1 (Thiamine)
In the United Kingdom deficiency is most commonly seen in alcoholism and presents with peripheral neuropathy or cardiomyopathy. Levels are not easy to measure and deficiency is assessed from:
1. Transketolase activity — heparinized whole blood.
   Normal 9–12 μmol/h per ml whole blood.

2. Urinary thiamine — normal 28–55 μmol/mol creatinine (higher in children).
3. Pyruvate studies — thiamine deficiency impairs pyruvate decarboxylation, raising the blood level. The tolerance test is more sensitive than serum levels.
4. A clinical response to thiamine 10 mg i.m. 8-hourly for 48 hours.

Blood Pyruvate

Normal
Heparinized whole blood

45–80 μmol/l

Samples must be taken with a cooled syringe, without a cuff or arm exercise, while the patient is fasting and resting. They are then immediately put into a special tube provided by the laboratory.

Increase
1. Physiological — after exertion and glucose.
2. Vitamin B_1 deficiency — beri-beri, alcoholism.
3. Poisoning — heavy metals.
4. Organ failure — cardiac, hepatic, renal, diabetic.

Pyruvate Metabolism Test
Glucose 75 g is given as for a glucose tolerance test (p. 124). Blood is taken at 30 and 60 minutes and the normal pyruvate level is not more than 100 μmol/l in both samples. An excessive prolonged rise (>150 μmol/l) is seen in:

1. Vitamin B_1 deficiency.
2. Heavy metal poisoning — not corrected by vitamin B_1.
3. Vitamin B_{12} deficiency with subacute combined degeneration of the cord.

Vitamin C (Ascorbic Acid)

Normal
Heparinized whole blood; sample to be taken rapidly the laboratory.

Plasma	45– 80 μmol/l
Buffy coat	114– 284 nmol/10^8 leucocytes
Pure leucocyte preparation	60–120 mmol/10^8 leucocytes

Saturation tests
1. Oral — the bladder is emptied at 8.00 a.m. and vitamin C 1 g is given. All urine is then collected until 11.00 a.m. The procedure is repeated daily until the ascorbic acid content of the three-hour collection exceeds 280 μmol (50 mg). This normally occurs by the second day. In mild deficiency it may take a week, and in clinical scurvy up to three weeks. In malabsorption urinary excretion may not reach this level.
2. Intravenous — vitamin C 500 mg is given i.v. and the urine collected for four hours. Normally over 40% of the dose is excreted, but less than 5% in frank scurvy. This test can be used in malabsorption.

Scurvy may present as a bleeding tendency in elderly or mal-nourished people. Plasma levels are unreliable and may be low in apparently normal people, perhaps due to temporary dietary deficiency. Values below 10 μmol/l are suggestive of scurvy. Leucocyte levels fall more gradually and indicate clinical deficiency more reliably. The saturation tests though criticized may be usefully combined with one of the blood levels.

Protein–calorie Malnutrition
Several measurements are available, none of which is ideal.

Height and weight
A weight below 80% of that expected for height is suggestive. In children a height below 90% of that expected for age is abnormal. In adults the weight–height index (W/H^2) should be between 20 and 25, where W = weight (kg) and H = height (m).

Skinfold thickness
Measurements are taken at several sites using a special caliper. At the mid triceps level the thickness should be over 5 mm in adult males and over 10 mm in adult females. This is a measurement of body fat.

Arm circumference

This measures muscle mass. It should be over 22 cm at the mid triceps level. Arm muscle circumference can be more accurately assessed by allowing for skinfold thickness.

Blood measurements

Serum transferrin, serum albumin and absolute lymphocyte counts are low.

Protein Loss

Daily nitrogen excretion = urinary urea (g/24 h) $\times$ 28/60 $\times$ 5/4. The corrections adjust for the molecular weights of nitrogen (28) and urea (60) and also for the fraction of nitrogen excreted as urea (4/5). In renal failure, daily protein catabolism can be calculated from the equation

Protein catabolism = Urinary urea (g/24 h $\times$ 3.5) + Serum urea rise (g/l $\times$ 1.8) $\times$ Body weight (kg) + Urine protein (g/24 h).

Chapter Seven

BACTERIAL INFECTION

Living organisms are divided into the eukaryotes: fungi, protozoa, and metazoa; and the prokaryotes: bacteria and viruses. Eukaryotes have a discrete nucleus with a nuclear membrane, but prokaryotes do not. Viruses contain either DNA or RNA, but bacteria contain both nucleic acids. Bacteria are classified as cocci (round in shape) or bacilli (long), as Gram positive (retaining blue dye) or Gram negative (staining pink). They may be aerobic and require oxygen to grow or anaerobic and require its absence. Facultative anaerobes grow less well without oxygen.

Full identification of bacteria, however, depends on other characteristics. Antibiotic sensitivity tests are of obvious clinical importance and may be more relevant than exact identification. Some bacteria are naturally resistant to certain antibiotics, e.g. pseudomonas to ampicillin. Resistance may also be acquired, e.g. staphylococci to benzylpenicillin. This is an especial problem with infections acquired in hospital.

DIAGNOSIS

The identification of an infecting organism is made by Gram staining and microscopy of infected material, by culture, by serology and by biochemical tests. Biochemical tests usually involve the identification of metabolites by colour reactions in the medium. The appearance of colonies and requirements for growth in culture are important means of identification.

Microscopy
The presence of infection may be confirmed by the finding of pus cells and organisms in secretions. Gram-staining may allow provisional identification of the species by an experienced observer, guiding immediate antibiotic treatment.

63

Culture

Specimens should be taken to the laboratory as soon as possible. A good sample of pus or exudate is the best culture source. Swabs should be premoistened with sterile water and sent in a transport medium. False-positives occur when a commensal or contaminant is treated as a pathogen. Contamination of normally sterile fluids like blood and CSF must be avoided by cleaning the skin with iodine and alcohol. It is important to know which organisms cause what sort of infection at any particular site because according to circumstances an organism may be either a commensal, pathogen or contaminant. Also, the bacteriologist must be told the source of the material, the clinical diagnosis and the antibiotic treatment given. Full identification of an organism with sensitivities takes 1–3 days. In severe infections of uncertain cause cultures must be taken from as many sites as possible, including blood and urine and, when relevant, the throat for streptococci and diphtheria, the faeces for enteric fever, and the vagina for toxic shock syndrome.

Serology

Antibodies appear in the blood in acute infection about 7–14 days after the onset of symptoms. A single high titre could be due to previous infection, particularly in patients from an endemic area, or to an anamnestic reaction, a non-specific rise caused by a different illness. A fourfold rise in titre during an illness is good evidence of active disease, so the first sample should be taken as soon as possible to provide a baseline. This means that in acute disease definite serological diagnosis may only be possible in retrospect. A negative result after several weeks rules out that infection. As IgM antibodies do not persist for long after acute infection, their presence is suggestive of active disease, whereas IgG antibodies may remain for some time after infection; this distinction is helpful, particularly in rubella and brucellosis.

Skin Testing

This demonstrates hypersensitivity and therefore present or past infection, e.g. tuberculin testing.

GRAM-POSITIVE COCCI

The Gram-positive cocci may sometimes be provisionally identified by Gram stain and microscopy of exudate. Staphylococci occur in clusters, streptococci in chains and pneumococci typically in pairs.

Streptococci
This heterogeneous group of organisms is differentiated by a combination of features, including type of haemolysis on blood agar, antigenic composition, growth characteristics and biochemical reactions.

Type of haemolysis
1. Beta-haemolytic — complete haemolysis giving a clear zone round the colony. The more virulent streptococci.
2. Alpha-haemolytic — partial or greenish haemolysis. Upper respiratory tract aerobic commensals.
3. Non-haemolytic — gastrointestinal organisms.

Antigenic structure
Streptococci are classified into Lancefield groups by precipitation with a specific antiserum which reacts with their cell-wall polysaccharide.

Group A. Str. pyogenes. For epidemiological work this group is divided into Griffith's types by surface antigens. Immunity to infection is specific to each type. Only some types are nephritogenic.

Group B. Beta-haemolytic streptococci causing perinatal sepsis and meningitis, subacute bacterial endocarditis (SBE) and urinary tract infection.

Group D. Usually non-haemolytic bowel organisms causing subacute bacterial endocarditis and urinary tract infection.

Non-groupable. Alpha-haemolytic organisms (*Str. viridans*) — the main cause of subacute bacterial endocarditis. Also anaerobic, often non-haemolytic organisms, causing abscesses.

Serology
Streptolysin-O is an oxygen labile haemolysin produced by beta-haemolytic streptococci. Antibody to it, antistreptolysin-O (ASO) appears within 1–2 weeks of infection, reaches a maximum of 3–5

weeks and disappears within 6–12 months. Normal levels in adults are below 166 U/ml and in school children they are below 330 U/ml. A fourfold rise in titre is diagnostic of recent infection. If titres never rise above 50 U/ml, this provides evidence against recent infection and therefore against rheumatic fever. In single samples of serum titres positive at very high dilution are also suggestive of recent infection. Skin infections are less often associated with high ASO titres than throat infections. The early use of antibiotics may prevent a rise in ASO titre. Griffith's type 12 infection, which may give rise to glomerulonephritis, does not always cause a rise in ASO titre. False-positive ASO tests do occur.

When rheumatic fever is suspected it is important to obtain evidence of recent streptococcal infection and other antibodies, e.g. antideoxyribonuclease B, antistreptokinase and antihyaluronidase, may indicate the presence of streptococcal antigens. It is very likely that at least one of these will be positive in rheumatic fever.

Str. pyogenes

These are all Group A and beta-haemolytic. They are identified in the laboratory by their sensitivity to bacitracin or by a fluorescent antibody test. They cause throat, skin and wound infection and in acute infection serological tests are not helpful. Allergy to these organisms causes acute rheumatic fever and acute glomerulonephritis and here serological tests are often more useful than swabs and cultures.

Str. pneumoniae (pneumococcus)

They may be recognizable in infected secretions as lanceolate diplococci. They are nasopharyngeal commensals and cause lobar pneumonia, bronchopneumonia, exacerbations of chronic bronchitis, otitis media and meningitis.

They also cause alpha-haemolysis, but are facultative anaerobes. Virulent organisms possess a capsule and can be distinguished from commensals by the mucoid colonies they form. They may be typed by antibodies to specific capsular carbohydrate antigens and type 3 is very virulent. Identification and typing may be speeded by incubation with specific antiserum, which causes the capsule to swell.

Str. viridans

This is a normal throat organism, which causes subacute bacterial endocarditis (SBE), but rarely other infection. It is distinguished from *Str. pneumoniae* by biochemical tests, but classification is sometimes difficult and the label may include assorted alpha-haemolytic streptococci.

Str. faecalis
Enterococci are streptococci normally occuring in the bowel. Those belonging to Group D are called *Str. faecalis*, whatever type of haemolysis they show. They cause urinary infection, infection after intra-abdominal operation and SBE.

Staphylococci
These organisms form small clusters, pairs or short chains in pus smears and may be seen within leucocytes unlike other Gram-positive cocci.

Staph. aureus (Staph. pyogenes)
All this group coagulate human plasma (coagulase positive) and are potential pathogens. They are identified by the appearance of the colonies on agar and by biochemical tests, e.g. mannitol fermentation. These organisms typically produce pus and cause abscesses. They cause infection of skin and wounds, osteomyelitis, septic arthritis, acute bacterial endocarditis, pneumonia with abscess formation and empyema. When they multiply in food they produce a toxin which causes food poisoning. They are also commensals in the nose and skin, and hospital employees usually carry penicillin-resistant strains. Diabetics are especially sensitive to pulmonary and skin infection.

Staph. saprophyticus (albus, epidermidis, micrococcus)
This organism is a common cause of cystitis in young female outpatients. It can also infect indwelling cannulas and cause endocarditis.

GRAM-POSITIVE BACILLI

Aerobic pathogens in this group include *Corynebacterium diphtheriae*, which is responsible for diphtheria, and *Bacillus anthracis*, which causes anthrax. *Listeria* and *Erysipelothrix* are animal pathogens, but in humans the former can cause meningitis and septicaemia and the latter can cause skin infections.

The main anaerobic pathogens are the Clostridia. *Cl. welchii (perfringens)* is a gut commensal which can gain entry to wounds, producing cellulitis, gas gangrene and toxaemia. *Cl. tetani* is found especially in manured soil. It invades wounds and produces a potent neurotoxin which causes tetanus. *Cl. botulinum* typically multiplies in badly canned food and its neurotoxin causes neuromuscular blockade, especially bulbar palsy. Lactobacilli are widespread human commensals. It has been suggested that they may be responsible for the urethral syndrome.

FILAMENTOUS BACTERIA

These are Gram-positive organisms. Actinomycetes cause actinomycosis. *Nocardia* can cause a pulmonary infection mistaken for tuberculosis. *N. madurae* causes Madura foot.

GRAM-NEGATIVE COCCI

The major group is the neisseriae, which are aerobic. The group includes meningococci and gonococci, as well as upper respiratory tract commensals. Meningococci and gonococci appear on microscopy of Gram-stained pathological material, typically as kidney shaped pairs often inside pus cells.

N. meningitidis

The meningococcus causes epidemic and sporadic purulent meningitis. It also causes a severe primary septicaemia, in which endotoxic shock and acute adrenal failure may occur. It can be an upper respiratory tract commensal.

N. gonorrhoeae

The gonococcus infects mucous membranes especially the urethra and cervix but the rectum and pharynx can be involved. Salpingitis, arthritis and septicaemia can also occur. Infection is more frequently chronic and asymptomatic in females than in males. The infection is acquired sexually and evidence of other sexual diseases, especially syphilis, must be sought.

Discharge should be examined by direct microscopy for pus and Gram-negative intracellular diplococci. Swabs should also be taken from the urethra, upper part of the vagina, endocervix and anal canal. They may be plated directly onto a selective culture medium or put into a transport medium for early culture.

GRAM-NEGATIVE BACILLI

These are mainly aerobic organisms, but anaerobic Gram-negative bacilli are the major bowel commensals and their importance in disease has been recognized.

Haemophilus influenzae

This small bacillus is an upper respiratory tract commensal. In adults it is associated with infective exacerbations of chronic bronchitis. In children it is a dangerous invasive organism, causing acute epiglottitis and meningitis. In smears, pleomorphic Gram-negative coccobacilli are seen. Invasive infections may be associated with bacteraemia.

Brucella species

In the UK, disease is usually due to *Br. abortus* and occurs mainly in those who have occupational contact with cattle or dairy products. Acute brucellosis presents with fever, headache and sweating. Chronic brucellosis can be difficult to diagnose. Pyrexia, sweating, joint pains and depression are common, but the ESR may be normal. A leucocytosis is unusual, but neutropenia with lymphocytosis is suggestive. Definitive diagnosis is by blood culture, but this is most likely to be positive early in the illness. Culture is difficult and can be dangerous to laboratory staff. Results may take up to three weeks. Serology can be inconclusive. In difficult cases, bone marrow culture, liver biopsy for histology and culture, and a therapeutic trial with appropriate antibiotics are considered.

Serology

In acute illness both agglutination and complement fixation tests become positive after a week, with a high and rising titre. Titres of over 1:1000 are expected, but levels of over 1:320 may be significant. In chronic brucellosis the interpretation of serology is difficult. High titres without infection occur anyway in people in exposed occupations and are also seen after cholera vaccination. In chronic brucellosis, direct agglutination tests, mainly IgM, are likely to be negative, but complement fixation tests and indirect agglutination tests (Coombs'), mainly IgG, should remain positive. Titres may, however, be low. Positive titres below 1:20 may be seen in apparent normals.

Allergy to *Br. abortus* without infection is associated with symptoms after contact and a high IgE level. Occupationally exposed people may also have high antibody titres but symptoms due to other conditions.

Pseudomonas aeruginosa
This is an opportunistic organism which infects burnt skin, lungs or the urinary tract after antibiotic control of a primary invader, or infects patients with serious underlying disease such as diabetes or cystic fibrosis. Infection is usually acquired in hospital. It is resistant to many antibiotics and antiseptics. Organisms grown from sputum may be contaminants, but cultures from other fluids are more reliable.

Enterobacteria
Many different groups of bacteria are normal gut commensals. Enterobacteriaceae is a large family of Gram-negative bacilli. They all ferment glucose and are differentiated, sometimes with difficulty, by other biochemical reactions. *Salmonella* and *Shigella* occur primarily as pathogens and usually do not ferment lactose. The *Proteus* group is a gut commensal. It swarms over solid media. *Escherichia* and *Klebsiella* ferment lactose.

Salmonella species
Sal. typhi and *Sal. paratyphi* A, B and C cause enteric fever, a septicaemic illness known as typhoid or paratyphoid. This might be suggested by the combination of pyrexia, leucopenia and lymphocytosis or monocytosis in a patient who has recently been abroad. There are many other salmonellae, e.g. *Sal. typhimurium*, which usually cause enteritis without blood stream invasion. Sometimes they cause pyrexia and bacteraemia.

Culture
A definitive diagnosis of enteric fever is best based on a positive

culture, and several cultures of blood, urine and stool should be made. Blood is most likely to be positive in the first two weeks and stool after that. Identification by the laboratory may take a few days. It may be helpful to culture blood clot.

Widal test

Presumptive evidence of enteric fever can be based on this serological test. *Salmonella* suspensions differently prepared to contain the various antigens are agglutinated by serial dilutions of serum. There is a somatic (O) antigen, a flagellar (H) antigen and freshly isolated strains, especially of *Sal. typhi*, have a surface Vi (vi for virulence) antigen. The Vi-antigen is recognized by susceptibility to viral bacteriophage. O-agglutinins appear on about the tenth day of infection and a fourfold rise in titre is diagnostic. They remain high for only a few months after natural infection or typhoid vaccination. H-agglutinins appear later in disease and occur less reliably. They persist for years after immunization or infection. There may be an anamnestic rise in titre when other infections occur. They are more specific, however, for different species of *Salmonella*. In the UK, titres for *Sal. paratyphi* A and C up to 1:10 are accepted as 'normal'. With *Sal. typhi* and *Sal. paratyphi* B, H titres of 1:30 and O titres of 1:50 are accepted.

Escherichia coli

E. coli is the most frequent aerobic species in the bowel and in adults it is the commonest cause of urinary tract infection. It can cause intra-abdominal sepsis and can invade other sites in debilitated patients. It causes neonatal meningitis. Enteropathogenic strains are associated with traveller's diarrhoea and epidemic diarrhoea in infants.

Proteus species

These cause urinary tract and wound infection. Being resistant to most antibiotics, they may persist after other organisms have been killed, but they are not alone in this.

Klebsiella species

Klebsiella pneumoniae (Friedländer's bacillus) causes cavitating pneumonia, meningitis, otitis media and sinusitis. *Klebsiella aerogenes* causes urinary tract and wound infections, but in the sputum is usually just a commensal which appears when other organisms have been eradicated by antibiotics.

Vibrio species

V. cholerae is the organism of cholera. The El Tor strain has spread through Asia, Africa and even Southern Europe, causing the reappearance of the disease in these areas.

Campylobacter jejuni is a vibrio isolated from the faeces by culture on a selective medium. It is a common cause of diarrhoea which can be mild but also severe and bloodstained. Septicaemia can occur.

Legionella pneumophila

This is a water-borne organism which often causes epidemic disease. A severe pneumonia occurs with systemic symptoms, renal, hepatic, cerebral or gstrointestinal. The clinical picture is not specific and the diagnosis is made by detecting antibodies with an indirect fluorescent antibody test, although culture is possible.

ANAEROBIC INFECTION

Anaerobic organisms grow only under reduced oxygen tension. They are most likely to be isolated if the laboratory is informed of the possibility and pus is taken there immediately and swabs put into a transport medium. Pus in anaerobic infection often smells putrid and on microscopy many different organisms are seen. Anaerobic infection should be especially considered in intra-abdominal infection, and pelvic infection in the female. It is important to diagnose it because of its restricted antibiotic sensitivity, but it is not always necessary to diagnose exactly which species is involved.

Bacteroides species are commensal in the mouth, colon and vagina. They are commonly involved in anaerobic infection.

SPIROCHAETES

Treponema pallidum

The causative organism of syphilis is identified by clinical microscopy or serology, not by culture.

Microscopy

Dark ground examination of material from primary or secondary lesions may be diagnostic and it is the only method of making the diagnosis before the serological tests become positive.

Non-specific serological tests

These depend on reaction between an antibody in the serum, called reagin, and a non-specific lipid antigen (probably similar to a lipid in spirochaetes). Most used is the Venereal Disease Research Laboratory (VDRL) test, a quantitative flocculation test which becomes positive three to five weeks after the infection has been contracted. The rapid plasma reagin (RPR) test is a simplified form of the VDRL test which can give a result in the clinic in 20 minutes. The cardiolipin Wassermann reaction (CWR) is a complement fixation test.

False-positives occur with these tests for several reasons, including technical error. They are positive in all treponemal diseases such as yaws. Some people normally have high serum reagin titres. Acute biological false-positive reactions occur after various viral infections and after typhoid or yellow fever immunization. They last for up to six months. Chronic biological false-positive reactions last for many years and occur in autoimmune disease such as systemic lupus erythematosus or rheumatoid arthritis.

Specific serological tests

The absorbed fluorescent treponemal antibody (FTA) test is the first test to become positive three to four weeks after infection. It is carried out by reacting the serum after removal of group specific antibody with killed treponemes. The *Treponema pallidum* haemagglutination (TPHA) test is the last test to become positive. Red cells are agglutinated when mixed with fragmented treponemes and serum antibody. The specific tests are positive with non-venereal treponematoses.

Diagnosis

The VDRL, FTA and TPHA tests should all be carried out to reduce error. If all are negative, syphilis can only be present in the early primary stage. If all are positive, syphilis, untreated or recently treated, is present.

If only the FTA is positive, early primary syphilis is likely. An isolated positive VDRL is likely to be a false-positive. A positive TPHA only suggests treated syphilis. A positive VDRL and FTA occurs in primary syphilis. A positive TPHA and FTA occurs in late syphilis and treated syphilis. The other treponematoses are distinguished from syphilis by clinical means.

Positive titres are highest in the secondary stage. IgM antibodies appear before IgG. Rising titres suggest active disease. The specific tests can remain positive for life, even in treated patients, and the VDRL may remain positive if treatment is given late. Serology is positive in infants of syphilitic mothers, but titres fall in a few months unless there is congenital infection.

Neurosyphilis

A CSF specimen not contaminated with blood must be examined. A lymphocytosis, high protein and high IgG suggest disease activity. A negative TPHA and FTA exclude neurosyphilis. However, the TPHA and FTA can be positive in the CSF in adequately treated disease. False-negative VDRL tests are common but a VDRL titre of over 1:8 suggests active disease, as biological false-positives do not occur.

Leptospira icterohaemorrhagiae

This organism is discharged in the urine of rats and is responsible for Weil's disease. It is frequently an occupational disease. There is pyrexia, headache, conjunctivitis, jaundice and there may be nephritis or meningitis. A neutrophil leucocytosis with a left shift is usual. Liver function tests are abnormal. Darkfield examination of the blood may be positive. Blood (three drops in a liquid medium), CSF and urine are cultured. The CSF may show a pleocytosis, at first polymorphonuclear then lymphocytic, but a normal sugar. Complement fixation and agglutination tests start to become positive at seven days and may remain elevated for years. They are the most reliable diagnostic methods.

Leptospira canicola

This infection is contracted from dogs. Jaundice is less frequent than in Weil's disease. The diagnostic approach is similar.

MYCOBACTERIA

Mycobacterium Tuberculosis

Every attempt must be made to confirm the diagnosis by bacteriological or histological means. Tuberculin testing is also useful. Sometimes the diagnosis has to rest on clinical or radiological findings. A therapeutic trial with antituberculous drugs is likely to produce a response within two weeks, but radiological improvement may take longer. Early confirmation of infection may be obtained from smears of sputum and other fluids, but those from urine are less reliable because of saprophytic mycobacteria. An auramine fluorescent stain is supplemented by the Ziehl–Neelsen stain, in which the bacteria are not decolourized by acid or alcohol. Infection is always confirmed by culture, which takes a minimum of two weeks to be positive.

Several samples of early morning urine or sputum should be taken and sent to the laboratory promptly. Gastric aspirates, laryngeal swabs and faecal specimens may also be examined.

In miliary tuberculosis bone marrow aspirates may be positive. Histological evidence and culture material can be obtained from nodes and, in miliary TB, from liver or bone marrow (allowed to clot and fixed in formalin for histology).

Tuberculin test
A positive tuberculin test indicates active or previous tuberculosis or BCG vaccination. Active infection is suggested by a positive test in a young child or conversion from negative to positive. A negative test with stronger tuberculin solutions is evidence against tuberculosis, except in the following circumstances.
1. Active tuberculosis — very early, overwhelming, or miliary disease.
2. Old age and cachexia.
3. Drugs — steroids, immunosuppressants.
4. Chronic disease — e.g. lymphomas or sarcoidosis (in which there is usually a negative reaction to 10 TU).

Technique. An intradermal injection of 0.1 ml of Old Tuberculin (OT) or purified protein derivative (PPD). The weakest strength contains one tuberculin unit (TU) as 1:10 000 OT or 0.02 µg of PPD. Weak solutions may give false-negatives. Strong solutions may cause an excessive reaction if disease or marked immunity is present. Adults should be given a 10 TU dose. Children and anyone with ocular involvement should be given a 1 TU dose. If this is negative a stronger solution is used. A negative reaction to 100 TU is good evidence against tuberculosis in a relatively well non-febrile individual.

Interpretation. The area of palpable induration is read at 48 hours. Induration less than 5 mm in diameter is negative, and induration more than 10 mm in diameter, especially with vesiculation, is strong positive.

Mycobacterium leprae

The diagnosis is made either by finding acid- but not alcohol-fast bacilli in tissue juice from a skin incision or by finding anaesthetic skin and a thickened nerve. The lepromin skin test is not helpful.

MYCOPLASMAS

Mycoplasmas, unlike other bacteria, lack rigid cell walls, and culture is difficult, requiring enriched media for growth. *M. pneumoniae* (Eaton agent) is the main pathogen and is a cause of primary atypical pneumonia in young people. It can also cause myringitis, rashes and haemolytic anaemia. Cold agglutinins, which agglutinate Group-O red cells at 4°C, often appear in the second week, and though they are non-specific, their presence is suggestive if there is pneumonia. A titre of over 1:32, especially if rising, is significant. A complement fixation test for *M. pneumoniae* is helpful.

RICKETTSIAE

Rickettsiae are small bacteria that can only be cultured in tissue. Serological tests are therefore necessary for diagnosis. *R. prowazekii* causes epidemic typhus. It is recognized by the Weil–Felix reaction, in which serum antibodies cross react with antigens from a *Proteus* strain.

Coxiella burnetii causes acute pyrexial illness, often presenting as atypical pneumonia (p. 211), and also SBE. When cultured in chick embryos it passes from a phase 1 to a phase 2 state. In acute infection there is a fourfold rise in antibody to the phase 2 antigen at 10–14 days and this is detected by a complement fixation test. Antibody to phase 1 rises more slowly and indicates chronic infection. A titre of over 1:200 can confirm endocarditis.

CHLAMYDIAE

These small bacteria are obligatory intracellular parasites. *Chlamydia psittaci* causes ornithosis. *C. trachomatis* serotypes A, B and C cause trachoma, serotypes D to K cause oculogenital disease, and serotypes L1, L2 and L3 cause lymphogranuloma venereum. Chlamydial infection should also be considered in culture-negative endocarditis. Chlamydiae can be grown in tissue culture, but serological diagnosis is more usual. There are complement fixation and microimmunofluorescent tests. A rising titre of IgM antibody is particularly important.

CLINICAL SYNDROMES

Acute Infection
Fever is usual and occurs more easily in children than adults. It may be absent in the elderly, with overwhelming infection and in patients taking corticosteroids or salicylates. Bacterial infection usually causes a neutrophil leucocytosis with a left shift and toxic granulation. Viral infection often causes neutropenia and sometimes true lymphocytosis. Leucopenia may also be seen with typhoid and rickettsial infection, with severe infection and in the previously ill patient. The ESR usually rises after 48 hours and albumin, calcium, phosphorus and sodium levels may fall. It should be remembered that inflammatory processes other than infections can cause pyrexia, leucocytosis and a raised ESR.

Chronic Infection
Normochromic anaemia with monocytosis and increased plasma cells in the marrow are common.

Septicaemia
The total white cell count may be normal or even low with infection by Gram-negative organisms, but neutrophil abnormalities as above occur. A Gram-stain of the buffy coat may be positive. Three blood cultures, aerobic and anaerobic, are taken at short intervals from different veins, and urine and all other possible sites of infection are cultured before starting treatment. Septicaemia may present with hypotension or intravascular coagulation (p. 277).

Abscess
High pyrexial spikes occur, with returns to baseline which are brief (hectic fever) or prolonged (intermittent fever). The neutrophil count is often over 20×10^9/l.

Pyrexia of Unknown Origin

This may be defined as a pyrexia over 38.3°C at least once daily for two weeks, unexplained by investigation in hospital for one week. Anaemia, a high ESR and proteinuria are non-specific in this condition, but severe anaemia points to malignancy, and an ESR of over 100 mm/l per h suggests malignancy or connective tissue disease (p. 141) and persistent proteinuria or microscopic haematuria suggests renal involvement. A neutrophil leucocytosis is typical of pyogenic infection, but may be absent and occurs also with neoplasms. Repeated aerobic and anaerobic culture of blood, urine, sputum, stool and, later, bone marrow are undertaken, as are serological tests for typhoid, brucellosis, leptospirosis, Q-fever, viruses and toxoplasmosis. Plain X-ray of the chest and abdomen are mandatory. Specialized studies including biopsies depend on the information gained from repeated examination of the patient and the preliminary tests. Radiological study of the abdominal viscera will usually be undertaken. Among the infections, tuberculosis, abdominal and pelvic abscess, endocarditis and biliary disease are always considered. Common non-infectious causes include connective tissue disease, lymphomas and occult, e.g. renal, neoplasms.

If no cause can be discovered, one might then embark on one of the following courses, choosing the one suggested by the clinical circumstances: a trial of broad-spectrum antibiotic; antituberculous treatment; steroids. Laparotomy used to be considered but has been replaced by ultrasound examination and computerized tomography.

Subacute Bacterial Endocarditis

In the classical case, *Streptococcus viridans* attacks an abnormal valve in a patient with carious teeth. Often the cardiac condition is not previously known. Other organisms may attack normal valves as in enterococcal bacteraemia, following urethral instrumentation. Various bacteria and fungi may be responsible in patients with prosthetic heart valves or intravascular catheters and in drug addicts or those receiving corticosteroid, cytotoxic or antimicrobial drugs. Endocarditis must be suspected in anyone with a heart murmur and unexplained fever.

Pyrexia, anaemia and a raised ESR are usual, and embolic phenomena and microscopic haematuria are common. Repeated clinical examination for cardiac pathology and embolism is necessary. Echocardiography may show vegetations. Usually six blood cultures from different sites are taken at two-hour intervals before starting treatment. If antibiotics have been given previously, treatment may be delayed and cultures spaced over several days.

When blood cultures are negative, fastidious bacteria require special culture techniques and serological tests for *Coxiella*, *Chlamydia*, *Brucella* and fungal infection are undertaken.

Acute Diarrhoea

Dietary indiscretion, faecal impaction, drugs and food poisoning cause diarrhoea, as well as infection. Food poisoning is associated with organic or inorganic contaminants as well as bacterial toxins, e.g. staphylococcal. Infection is particularly suggested by pyrexia and recent travel.

Invasive organisms inflame the colonic mucosa and pus and blood is found on stool microscopy. This occurs with *Shigella* and *E. coli* and also with *Salmonella*, *E. histolytica* and *Campylobacter*. Pus does not occur when diarrhoea is due to enterotoxins, or with *Giardia* and some *Salmonella* and *E. coli*. Microscopy of the stool and the culture of fresh specimens are of primary importance and sigmoidoscopy is most useful in chronic diarrhoea.

Campylobacter jejuni is a common cause of sporadic acute diarrhoea. *Yersinia enterocolitica* affects the ileum and may cause an arthritis. *Giardia lamblia* (p. 88) can cause chronic diarrhoea. *Clostridium difficile* can cause antibiotic-associated colitis, which may be pseudomembranous in appearance. Ulcerative colitis may present with very acute bloody diarrhoea and it may be complicated by superadded infection.

In children, diarrhoea is usually viral, especially Rotaviruses in the infant, but *E. coli* is the commonest bacterial pathogen. In this age group, infections outside the gastrointestinal tract also cause diarrhoea.

Reduced Resistance to Infection

This situation is common in hospital practice. It occurs due to neutropenia, impaired antibody responses, or reduced cell-mediated immunity (CMI). Other factors such as the breach of epithelial barriers by instrumentation and antibiotic resistant organisms occurring in the hospital environment are important. Organisms of normally low pathogenicity, opportunists, may become invasive and cause atypical, severe, or disseminated infection.

Gram-negative organisms, such as *E. coli* and *Pseudomonas aeruginosa*, frequently attack patients with reduced CMI, as after transplantation, or those with neutropenia and they emerge after antibiotic use. Gram-positive organisms, such as *Staph. albus*, infect patients with i.v. or urethral catheters. Fungi, such as *Candida* and *Aspergillus*, attack patients after transplants or after chemotherapy for lymphoma.

Viruses, especially the herpes group (p. 83), attack similar patients. Protozoal infections, e.g. with *Pneumocystis carinii*, also occur after transplantation and are important. The sitution is iatrogenic. Sick people perforce receive treatment which reduces resistance to infection and they are also exposed to abnormal risks.

Chapter Eight

NON-BACTERIAL INFECTION

VIRUSES

Viruses are in general much smaller than bacteria and only the largest can be seen by light microscopy. They are intracellular parasites and can only be grown in tissue culture, not on inanimate laboratory media. They possess only a single type of nucleic acid, either DNA or RNA, and reproduce not by binary fission but after infecting a cell, by the virus particle breaking down and its nucleic acid synthesizing more virus-specific protein. They are not affected by antibiotics, though antiviral agents are becoming increasingly available.

Diagnosis

The three main methods used are electron microscopy, viral culture and serology.

Electron microscopy is helpful in gastroenteritis and vesicular skin rashes. Fluorescent microscopy using fluorescent antibody can be used in CSF and material from skin vesicles.

Viral culture is most likely to be positive in the early phase of an illness, but as tissue culture is necessary it is expensive, difficult and delayed. Secretions are more productive than swabs. Vesicles as in herpetic infection may be aspirated into a tuberculin syringe which is capped and sent to the laboratory. Any swabs should be rubbed against the lesion and sent at once in a transport medium to the laboratory. The cultured organism is recognized by the specific lesions it produces in tissue or by its neutralization by specific antibody.

Serological diagnosis

This may be positive early in the illness when specific IgM antibodies are present. Otherwise near diagnostic certainty that there is active rather than previous infection can only be achieved by a fourfold rise in titre between the first serum and one taken at least a week later. An initial negative does not exclude disease but a late one does. An initial positive may be due to past infection. The major tests are:

1. Complement fixation test (CFT).
2. Neutralization — the usual effects of the virus on tissue culture are prevented by serum antibody.
3. Haemagglutination-inhibition (HAI) — serum antibody prevents agglutination of red cells by viral antigen.

Rubella

Accurate diagnosis becomes important when a pregnant woman develops a suspicious illness or is in contact with a case. The diagnosis is serological and the contact case should be examined also.

Haemagglutination-inhibiting antibody (HAI test) appears within two days of the rash, peaks within two weeks, and persists. It is a reliable screening test, but its presence does not prove that infection is recent. IgM HAI antibody, however, disappears within eight weeks. Complement fixing antibodies (CFT) appear seven days after the rash, peak within two months and then decline. In difficult cases a combination of these tests, repeated after an interval, will indicate whether infection is recent. A positive HAI test in a well person indicates immunity and a negative test indicates susceptibility to infection. In the neonate, viral culture may be necessary as maternal antibody is present.

Viral Hepatitis

Acute hepatitis is frequently caused by virus A (infectious hepatitis) or virus B (serum hepatitis). In both forms transaminase levels are high and precede the appearance of jaundice. The rise in alkaline phosphatase is modest (p. 163). Leucopenia and lymphocytosis may occur. Virus A causes classical infectious hepatitis. Virus B hepatitis is less common and has a longer incubation period and a more insidious onset. Infection is acquired by contact with blood products or through sexual activity. A polyarthritis may occur. Hepatitis may be associated with other viruses such as Coxsackie, cytomegalovirus and infectious mononucleosis, as well as a not yet fully defined non-A, non-B hepatitis. Amoebiasis, malaria, septicaemia, tox-aemias and drugs cause non-viral hepatitis.

Hepatitis A
IgM antibody appears at the onset of the disease and persists for up to eight weeks. IgG antibody then appears and then persists for life. Its presence indicates immunity to infection with hepatitis A virus.

Hepatitis B
After infection by hepatitis B virus a surface antigen from the viral coat (HB$_s$Ag) is the first marker of disease to appear in the blood. Biochemical evidence of hepatitis then appears and during this phase anti-HBc, an antibody to a viral core antigen, appears. This is the most sensitive test for hepatitis B and its absence excludes the diagnosis. It persists for some time after recovery. With biochemical recovery HB$_s$Ag usually disappears and the antibody to it, anti-HB$_s$, appears. It persists and its presence usually indicates immunity to infection. A negative HB$_s$Ag test with a positive anti-HB$_c$ test is consistent with acute or previous hepatitis. If anti-HB$_s$ is present early in a disease acute hepatitis B is unlikely.

Chronic carriers of hepatitis B virus have persistent HB$_s$Ag in the blood. They are also anti-HB$_c$ positive. They are clinically well but usually have abnormal liver function tests and abnormal liver biopsies. This situation most commonly occurs in patients from underdeveloped areas, patients with impaired immunity, dialysis patients and sufferers from Down's syndrome. Positive HB$_s$Ag tests may also be associated with chronic active hepatitis, systemic vasculitis and glomerulonephritis. HB$_s$Ag is detected by various techniques including enzyme immunoassay (ELISA).

Herpes Viruses
This is a group of DNA viruses which produce intranuclear inclusion bodies in infected cells. They include herpes simplex, varicella-zoster virus, cytomegalovirus and Epstein–Barr virus.

Herpes Simplex
This causes aphthous stomatitis, genital infection, keratoconjunctivitis, meningitis and encephalitis. It attacks especially immunocompromised hosts. It can be cultured in tissue when the cells show inclusion bodies. Rising titres of complement fixing antibodies are associated with infection.

Cytomegalovirus

Infection in utero causes fetal malformation and neonatal illness. Adults may develop hepatitis, a glandular fever syndrome or PUO. At particular risk are adults affected by other severe chronic disease or treated by immunosuppressive drugs. In particular danger are women of child-bearing age working in special-care baby units. Diagnosis can be made by culture of urine or saliva and serological tests. Complement-fixing antibodies in a healthy person indicate previous infection, usually subclinical, and immunity to further infection.

Infectious Mononucleosis

Most cases are caused by the Epstein–Barr virus and have a positive Paul–Bunnell test. The clinical picture is variable and pyrexia, lymphadenopathy, sore throat or hepatitis may predominate. Over 50% of the white cells are lymphocytes or monocytes and over 20% of these are atypical. The Paul–Bunnell test may be persistently negative in up to 20% of cases and an experienced observer may base the diagnosis on a typical blood film and the clinical picture. However the presence of abnormal WBC alone is not sufficiently diagnostic and a negative test indicates consideration of other conditions such as toxoplasmosis and cytomegalovirus. It is especially important to exclude the latter two in pregnancy.

Paul–Bunnell test

Antibodies produced in infectious mononucleosis agglutinate sheep red cells. Non-speciic antibodies may be present which will also do so, but which can be absorbed by prior contact with an antigen in guinea pig kidney, whereas the true infectious mononucleosis antibody is absorbed by prior contact with ox red cells. The classical test using sheep cells and tube dilutions has been largely replaced by a slide test using horse cells. It is usually positive by the second week of the illness. False-positives can occur with malignant blood conditions and malaria.

FUNGAL INFECTIONS

Fungi are mainly saprophytic plants which differ from bacteria in their morphology, mode of reproduction and insensitivity to antibacterial antibiotics.

They are divided into:

1. Yeasts — which are round or oval bodies, reproducing by buds.
2. Moulds — whose filaments form a tangled mass, a mycelium.
3. Dimorphic fungi — which are like typical yeasts in their parasitic phase and like moulds when they are grown as saprophytes.

Infection by fungi is a mycosis. In the United Kingdom, cutaneous mycoses are much commoner than systemic mycoses. Fungi, especially *C. albicans*, cause opportunistic infections. They invade patients whose resistance is affected by disease such as leukaemia or diabetes or by drugs such as antibiotics or immunosuppressants.

Diagnosis

Direct microscopy of skin scrapings, hair and nail clippings is commonly sufficient. Digestion of keratin by 20% NaOH may be helpful. Culture on an acidic glucose agar medium (Sabouraud) is not difficult but slow. Serological tests and skin tests for delayed hypersensitivity are useful in systemic mycoses. Antibodies, however, occur in healthy people who may also have positive skin tests to the commoner fungi which they are likely to have previously met.

Yeasts

These include *Cryptococcus neoformans*, which causes chronic meningitis, and *Candida albicans*.

Candida albicans

C. albicans is a common cause of skin and nail infection, vaginitis and stomatitis. Other candidal species are less frequently seen. Treatment with antibiotics and steroids, immunodeficiency, hypoparathyroidism, diabetes and hypoadrenalism predispose to infection.

Systemic candidiasis is not common. Candidae appear in the sputum after antibiotics, but this does not imply tissue invasion, nor does the presence of candida in the urine unless the concentration is over 10^4/ml. Candida sepsis and septicaemia may be related to indwelling cannulae and artificial heart valves. The organism may be recognized on a smear or by culture.

Moulds

Fungi of the genera *Microsporum*, *Trichophyton* and *Epidermophyton* cause ringworm or tinea. Members of the genus *Aspergillus* can cause systemic infection.

Aspergillus fumigatus

A. fumigatus causes aspergillosis. One manifestation is allergic pulmonary aspergillosis, characterized by asthma, pulmonary infiltration and collapse, and eosinophilia in sputum and blood. A saprophytic form can cause mycetomas in old tuberculous cavities or may become invasive especially in a compromised host.

Diagnosis is based on the total picture. Fresh sputum is examined and cultured, but if the organism is only isolated once it could be a contaminant. Positive skin tests and a high IgE level provide helpful evidence in the allergic type and serum precipitins in all types of infection.

Dimorphic Fungi

These include *Histoplasma capsulatum*, which mainly attacks the lung. The diagnosis can be confirmed by immunodiffusion and complement fixation tests. The organism can also be demonstrated in the sputum in cavitating disease.

PROTOZOA

Protozoa are unicellular organisms with an organization like that of animal cells and which often have complex life cycles. The more severe infections occur mainly outside the temperate zones. The Sporozoa include the plasmodia, *Toxoplasma gondii*, and *Pneumocystis carinii*. *Giardia lamblia* and *Trichomonas vaginalis* are intestinal flagellates and *Trypanosoma cruzi* and *Leishmania donovani* are flagellates which invade the blood. Amoebae such as *Entamoeba histolytica*, and ciliate forms like *Balantidium coli* also cause disease.

Entamoeba histolytica

This parasite exists as a vegetative form (trophozoite), which lives in the colon often as a commensal, and as a cyst, which can survive outside the body and infect others. It causes dysentery and hepatic abscess. Colonic amoebiasis is diagnosed by the finding of amoeboid trophozoites with ingested red cells. These can be found best in mucus from a lesion seen on sigmoidoscopy, but are usually found by microscopy of warm freshly passed stools. Saline purges may be used to produce loose stools but no other laxatives or enemas should be used and there should be no barium in the specimen. Cysts may sometimes be found in a saline emulsion of firm stools but do not indicate active disease.

Amoebic liver abscess presents with pain, pyrexia, local tenderness, leucocytosis and evidence of a space-occupying lesion shown by available imaging techniques.

Serology
The complement fixation and fluorescent antibody tests are sensitive. Latex agglutination and immunodiffusion tests are rapid and cheap. Tests tend to remain positive after recovery, but the gel diffusion precipitation test reverts to negative. Serology is reliable in liver abscess but less so in colonic disease, where it is still useful with amoebomas and in the distinction from ulcerative colitis.

Malaria
This diagnosis must be considered in anyone with pyrexia or other obscure illness who has recently visited or passed through a malarious area. Of the four main species of malarial parasite, *Plasmodium falciparum* is the most dangerous, but symptoms usually present within two weeks of exposure. It must be considered as a cause of coma, acute renal failure and hepatic failure. *P. malariae* may be the most difficult to diagnose when parasitaemia is of low density and intermittent. *P. vivax* has an incubation period up to nine months.

An experienced observer should see a thick blood film to discover the parasite and a standard thin blood film to identify the species. In early illness, films may be taken at four-hour intervals until parasitaemia is sufficiently heavy for recognition. Serial films may also be necessary in chronic *P. malariae* infection. In the latter case serodiagnostic tests may be especially helpful but are not widely available.

Toxoplasma gondii
Humans are infected by cat faeces or uncooked meat. Infection is most serious when acquired in pregnancy and causes congenital toxoplasmosis. Stillbirth, choroiditis, hydrocephalus, cerebral calcification and other brain damage may result.

Serology
Haemagglutination, latex agglutination, dye tests and ELISA tests are available. Positive tests at low titre are common and usually indicate past infection. Titres are not usually high, however, in active ocular toxoplasmosis. High and rising titres suggest active systemic disease. Positive tests in infants at six months are likely to be significant.

Trichomonas vaginalis
The male is usually asymptomatic, as may be the female, who typically has vaginitis. Other venereal diseases may be associated. Material is taken from vagina, cervix and urethra. Recognition is on a wet unstained film, or by dark ground illumination, by Papanicolaou stain or by culture from Stuart's medium.

Giardia lamblia
Diarrhoea and malabsorption may occur. Jejunal oedema may be shown by X-ray. Trophozoites may be found in loose stools. Cysts are sought in formed stools by staining after concentration with formol ether. If several stools are negative the trophozoite may be found in jejunal fluid, a smear made from a jejunal biopsy or in the stained biopsy specimen.

METAZOA (PARASITES)

Schistosomiasis (Bilharziasis)
Eosinophilia with haematuria or diarrhoea is suggestive of urinary or intestinal involvement. Diagnosis is by finding eggs in urine, stool, or mucosal biopsy. An endstream urine specimen collected at midday is best. If a stool suspension is exposed to light, miracidia may hatch out and be seen by naked eye. Rectal biopsy may demonstrate eggs and i.v. urography may show suggestive lesions. A complement fixation test is possible.

Intestinal Worms
Diagnosis in each case depends on the examination of fresh stools. Hookworm causes iron deficiency anaemia and roundworms cause vague abdominal symptoms. All worms can cause eosinophilia, especially hookworm.

Trichinella spiralis

Spread of larvae through the body causes muscle pains, fever and marked eosinophilia, sometimes also periorbital oedema. Muscle biopsy from the thigh is usually positive. Serological tests are possible.

Echinococcus granulosus

In hydatid disease, cystic tumours of liver, lung or brain with eosinophilia and sometimes calcification occur. Complement fixation and haemagglutination tests are available.

Chapter Nine

THYROID DISEASE

Physiology

Ingested iodide is taken up by the thyroid gland, oxidized to organic iodine and incorporated into tyrosine. Iodinated tyrosine compounds combine to form thyroxine (T4) with four iodine molecules. Non-thyroid tissue converts T4 into tri-iodothyronine (T3) by removal of an iodine molecule. This is present in much smaller quantity than T4 but is much more active. T4 can be converted into inactive reverse T3 by the removal of a different iodine molecule. Thyroxine stimulates oxygen consumption in all tissues. Thyrotrophin-releasing hormone (TRH) from the hypothalamus stimulates pituitary thyroid stimulating hormone (TSH) production, which increases thyroid T4 synthesis. Raised free T4 and T3 levels suppress pituitary TSH production.

Circulating Hormones

Measurement of serum T4, T3 and TSH is the basis of the study of thyroid activity. T4 and T3 are largely bound to a carrier protein, thyroxine-binding globulin (TBG). TBG is normally about 30% saturated. Changes in TBG concentration and binding ability affect the serum total thyroxine (TT4) and total tri-iodothyronine (TT3) concentrations. TT4 and TT3 levels must be interpreted in conjunction with an assessment of TBG binding capacity. It is the free hormone that is biologically active and direct measurement of free T4 and T3 is preferable.

Serum Free Thyroxine (FT4)

Normal
8.8–23.2 pmol/l

This measurement is replacing the TT4 and avoids the problems caused by changes in TBG concentration and T4 binding. Measurement requires a preliminary dialysis of the serum. An increase is seen in hyperthyroidism and in hypothyroidism treated by thyroxine (p. 97). A decrease is seen in hypothyroidism. Fluctuations in the FT4 level occur with illness and drugs, as explained below.

Serum Free Tri-iodothyronine (FT3)

Normal

Adults	3.0–8.6 pmol/l
Infants	5.5–7.0 pmol/l

The FT3 concentration usually parallels that of FT4, but sometimes in thyrotoxicosis T3 levels are preferentially raised and it is better to measure both FT3 and FT4 in cases of doubt.

High FT3 levels with normal FT4

In up to 5% of hyperthyroid patients the FT4 may be normal despite a raised T3, e.g.

1. T3 thyrotoxicosis — sometimes seen in early or relapsing disease.
2. Endocrine exophthalmos.
3. Thyroid nodules.
4. Iodine deficiency.
5. Carbimazole treatment.

Low FT3 levels with normal FT4

In certain circumstances there is reduced conversion of T4 to T3. The patients are not hypothyroid but have a 'euthyroid sick syndrome'.

1. Illness — all catabolic diseases, especially hepatic disease and starvation.
2. Drugs — iodinated compounds, e.g. biliary contrast media and amiodarone; glucocorticoids, propranolol, propylthiouracil.

Serum Total Thyroxine (TT4)

Total plasma T4 is measured by immunoassay which detects the bound T4 as well as the small fraction of biologically active unbound T4.

Normal

Adults	64–142 nmol/l
Neonates	125–270 nmol/l

Infants & children	85–190 nmol/l
Elderly	60–140 nmol/l
Pregnancy	80–220 nmol/l

Increase
1. Thyrotoxicosis.
2. High TBG — this occurs in pregnancy and is rarely congenital. Oestrogens including the contraceptive pill raise TBG levels. A rise may also occur in liver disease and acute porphyria.
3. Thyroxine treatment.

Decrease
1. Hypothyroidism.
2. Low TBG — this occurs in illnesses likely to lower serum albumin levels, such as nephrotic syndrome, hepatic failure and malnutrition. It is rarely congenital. It may be caused by androgens and corticosteroids.
3. Reduced binding of T4 by TBG — this occurs in renal failure, liver failure and diabetic coma. T4-binding is reduced by aspirin, iodine and phenytoin.

Serum Total Tri-iodothyronine (TT3)

Normal

| Adults | 1.8–3.1 nmol/l |
| Infants | 1.5–4.0 nmol/l falling to adult values by the age of 15 years. |

TT3 levels, like FT3 levels, are affected by T4 production and T4-to-T3 conversion. They are also affected by changes in TBG concentration and binding capacity.

Thyroid Hormone Binding Tests

These tests measure the number of unoccupied binding sites on the serum TBG. They are necessary to correctly interpret TT4 and TT3 levels if there is any possibility of a change in the thyroxine binding globulin (TBG) level or of an abnormal substance binding to it. A known quantity of radioactive T3 is added to a mixture of test serum and an inert T3 acceptor (e.g. resin). The T3 partitions between the acceptor and the serum TBG, according to the number of free binding sites in the serum. If the serum activity is measured as in the 'Thyopac-3' test, low values indicate few free binding sites (normal 92–117). The reverse applies if the resin is measured as in some methods, e.g. 'Trilute'. Although it is a T3 uptake (T3U) test it must not be confused with T3 measurement.

Increased free binding sites occur when the TBG level is high and in hypothyroidism because TBG is less saturated. Decreased free binding sites occur when TBG is low, has a reduced T4-binding capacity and in thyrotoxicosis when TBG is more saturated.

Free Thyroxine Index (FTI)

Normal
Adults   5.5–10.0
Neonates   9–26, falling gradually to adult values by the age of six years.

The FTI is derived from the TT4 and the measurement of free T4-binding sites (T3U). It correlates with the FT4 level but is less reliable.

$$FTI = TT4 \times \frac{Control\ T3U}{Patient\ T3U}$$

In thyrotoxicosis, TT4 is high and T3U is low, so the FTI is high. In pregnancy, TT4 is high and T3U is high, so FTI is normal. If the resin not the serum activity is measured in the test available, the equation becomes

$$FTI = TT4 \times \frac{Patient\ T3U}{Control\ T3U}$$

PITUITARY–THYROID AXIS TESTS

The axis is assessed by measurement of TSH and its stimulation by thyrotrophin-releasing hormone.

Serum Thyroid Stimulating Hormone (TSH)

Normal
Below 6 mIU/l

Measurement by radioimmunoassay is not sensitive enough to distinguish low from normal levels.

Increase
1. Primary hypothyroidism — a normal TSH level excludes primary thyroid failure.
2. Other thyroid disease — a moderate rise in serum TSH (< 20 mU/l) is seen in euthyroid patients with goitres, Hashimoto's disease and after treatment of hyperthyroidism by drugs, surgery or radiation. Some but not all of these patients become hypothyroid later.

Thyrotrophin-releasing Hormone (TRH) Test
TSH is measured before and 20 and 60 minutes after synthetic TRH 200 μg i.v. Thyroxine and corticosteroids must be avoided before the test. There should normally be a rise of at least 2 mIU/l to above normal, but not above 20 mIU/l. The level is maximal at 20 minutes.

Increased response
1. Primary hypothyroidism — it is the most sensitive test.
2. Drugs — oestrogens.

Reduced response
1. Thyrotoxicosis — a normal response excludes it but a reduced response does not confirm it.
2. Other thyroid disease — goitres, adenomas and endocrine exophthalmos, even if euthyroid.
3. Pituitary disease — a normal response excludes secondary hypothyroidism. A reduced response is seen in about 50% of patients with pituitary disease but does not necessarily imply a need for thyroxine. In hypothalamic disease the 20 minute level may be low and the 60 minute level is typically higher.
4. Other disease — chronic renal failure, endogenous depression.
5. Drugs — thyroxine, corticosteroids, levodopa.

RADIOISOTOPE TESTS

Radioactive Iodine Uptake (RAIU)

Neck counts are determined after an oral dose of isotope. ^{131}I is used most commonly and measurements are made at six hours for hyperthyroidism and at 24 hours for hypothyroidism. It is more reliable for hyperthyroidism than for hypothyroidism, but is much less used now. Some people use it to assess the dose for radioiodine treatment. In atypical thyrotoxicosis a low uptake may point to thyroiditis, or administration of iodine or thyroxine.

Increase (> 30%)
1. Thyrotoxicosis.
2. Iodine deficiency.

Decrease (< 15%)
1. Hypothyroidism.
2. Iodine administration.
3. Thyroxine — sometimes taken secretly.
4. Abnormal metabolism — congenital or induced by antithyroid drugs.
5. Acute thyroiditis (p. 97).

Other isotopes
^{132}I is sometimes used because of the reduced radiation dose and because the test can be repeated next day. A 20-minute uptake after i.v. technetium is a convenient screening test for hyperthyroidism, which is not affected by antithyroid treatment, as technetium uptake reflects iodine trapping and antithyroid drugs inhibit iodine organification.

Thyroid Scans
The uses of the scan are as follows:
1. The solitary nodule — a 'hot' nodule is not malignant, but a 'cold' nodule can be (p. 98).
2. Ectopic tissue — functioning metastases and normal ectopic tissue may be located.

Thyroid Antibodies
Thyroid antimicrosomal antibodies and antithyroglobulin antibodies

are usually detected. With the former, titres of 1:100 are considered positive. The tests are now usually performed with a tanned red cell haemagglutination method in which the cells are coated with antigen before exposure to test serum.

Uses
1. Suspected thyroid disease — the presence of thyroid antibodies provides some confirmation. This can be useful in endocrine exophthalmos and doubtful hypothyroidism.
2. Autoimmune thyroiditis — the higher the levels in a patient with goitre, the more likely is the diagnosis. Antibody levels rise before hypothyroidism appears.

Weak positive tests can occur in apparently normal people, various autoimmune conditions and all thyroid diseases.

Tests of Tissue Response
These are too non-specific to be diagnostic, but changes can be useful in monitoring the response to a trial of treatment in doubtful cases.

Electrocardiogram
In hypothyroidism, amplitude of the R and T waves may decrease and reversion to normal is some evidence of response to treatment.

Serum cholesterol
Serum cholesterol tends to rise in hypothyroidism and fall in thyrotoxicosis but it is not a useful clinical test.

Reflex relaxation time
Though this can be measured, clinical evidence of slow relaxation of the ankle jerks is sufficient. It is a useful screening test for hypothyroidism, but non-specific.

CLINICAL PROBLEMS

Hyperthyroidism: Diagnostic Problems
However clear the clinical picture, a T4 level and a test of thyroid hormone binding capacity or a free T4 level is taken off before treatment is started. T3 measurement is indicated only if there is doubt after T4 measurement. This may occur in circumstances that

affect T4 concentration (p. 91) or in borderline cases. If there is still doubt, an abnormal TRH test justifies a trial of carbimazole.

Ongoing treatment
To assess the adequacy of drug treatment it is necessary to measure both T4 and T3 concentrations. T3 levels are relatively high with carbimazole treatment. The T3 level should be normal and the T4 level on the low side. If the TSH level rises, the patient has been overtreated. Weight changes and heart rate are two good clinical guides.

Pregnancy
In normal pregnancy there is a high cardiac output and a small goitre may appear. Also total T4 rises because of the rise in TBG and isotope tests must be avoided. Assessment is therefore difficult. Drugs must be used cautiously because of their goitrogenic effect on the fetus and the tendency of the condition to remit in the third trimester. Tests return to normal by ten weeks postpartum.

Viral thyroiditis
This may cause temporary thyrotoxicosis and a raised T4 due to acute hormone release. There is usually pain and radioactive iodine uptake is low. The ESR is high.

Hypothyroidism: Diagnostic Problems
Before treatment is started blood is taken for a T4 level and for an FTI or a free T4 level and also for a TSH level.

Doubtful hypothyroidism
In the presence of suggestive symptoms and a borderline T4 value, a raised TSH level favours a trial of treatment. A normal TSH level excludes primary hypothyroidism, but pituitary disease might be considered. If the TSH level is borderline, an enhanced TRH response favours the use of thyroxine.

Ongoing treatment
Assessment of improvement is essentially clinical, but the TSH level will fall to normal after two months on adequate treatment and the tests of tissue response (p. 96) may change. The T4 level is slightly high and the T3 level is normal with adequate replacement.

Endocrine Exophthalmos

Unilateral exophthalmos without a local cause presents a difficult problem in the absence of obvious thyrotoxicosis. It is helpful to confirm a suspected diagnosis of endocrine exophthalmos in bilateral and unilateral cases by finding some evidence of thyroid disease. Thyroid antibodies may be present or the TRH test may be abnormal. Computed tomography helps to exclude a tumour.

Goitre

The two main questions asked are whether the patient is euthyroid and whether there is a possibility of neoplasm. Relevant tests include ESR, T4, T3, TSH, antibodies and a scan.

Diffuse goitre

A neoplasm is suspected if the gland is fixed, hard or enlarging rapidly. In Hashimoto's disease, thyroid antibodies are present and there may be hypothyroidism or at least a raised TSH level. The ESR may be high and other autoimmune diseases may coexist. Other causes of diffuse non-toxic goitre are iodine deficiency, goitrogen ingestion including antithyroid drugs, and enzyme defects. Any suspicion of malignancy is an indication for surgical referral.

Nodular goitre

With multinodular glands, treatment is indicated only for thyrotoxicosis or pressure symptoms. With single nodules, if a scan shows hypofunction ('cold nodule'), neoplasm, cyst, and thyroiditis are considered. Ultrasound examination, needle aspiration of a cyst for cytology and surgical referral are appropriate.

Drugs and the Thyroid

The effects of drugs on thyroid binding globulin levels, binding of T4 and T4-to-T3 conversion are indicated above. Goitre and hypothyroidism may be caused by drugs that interfere with iodine metabolism, including: carbimazole and allied drugs, PAS, excess iodine (usually in cough mixtures and asthma remedies), lithium, phenylbutazone, resorcinol, and possibly sulphonylureas and phenothiazines, though the effect is not great. Iodine and thyroxine ingestion cause thyrotoxicosis. Propranolol improves the symptoms of thyrotoxicosis.

Chapter Ten

ADRENAL DISEASE

The adrenal cortex secretes cortisol, aldosterone and androgens. The syndromes caused by excess or deficiency of these hormones are defined by studying the hormones and their metabolites in blood and urine. Urine tests are mainly useful in the study of glandular hyperfunction, as excretion is reduced in many illnesses. Further information is obtained by dynamic tests in which the effects of stimulation and suppression on hormone secretion are analysed.

IMAGING

Plain abdominal X-ray may reveal calcification. Computerized tomography may detect an adenoma or hyperplasia.

URINE AND PLASMA HORMONES

Serum Cortisol

Normal
9.00 a.m. (fasting)	330–770 nmol/l
11.00 p.m.	110–390 nmol/l

Measurement is by radioimmunoassay, which has replaced fluorescence methods. Prednisolone and oestrogen interfere with the assay.

Increase
1. Cushing's syndrome of all causes.
2. Cortisol-binding globulin (CBG)—the carrier protein is increased in pregnancy and with oestrogens. Free cortisol and biological activity (compare thyroid-binding globulin) is not affected.
3. Stress—acute anxiety, chronic stress, hypoglycaemia, chronic alcoholism, depressive disorders.
4. Miscellaneous—obesity, hyperthyroidism.

Decrease
1. Adrenal failure—Addison's disease, congenital adrenal hyperplasia, hypopituitarism.
2. Hypothyroidism.
3. Liver disease.

Urine Free Cortisol

Normal

Adult males	300–1100 nmol/24 h
Adult females	215– 860 nmol/24 h
Early morning urine	50– 550 nmol cortisol per 10 mmol creatinine.

An increase is seen in Cushing's disease and pregnancy. Measurement is not helpful in the diagnosis of adrenal hypofunction. Values depend on the method of estimation and the individual laboratory.

Urine 17-Oxosteroids (17-OS)

Normal

Adult males	20–70 μmol per 24 h; females 16–52 μmol per 24 h
Children	show a gradual rise towards adult levels.
Elderly	excretion falls after age 50.
Pregnancy	a rise by 50%.

It is a colorimetric assay affected by drugs, including tranquillizers and antibiotics. 17-OS are derived largely from adrenal steroid precursors, with lesser amounts from the testes and ovaries. Elevation is seen with Cushing's syndrome, especially when it is due to adrenal carcinoma, with congenital adrenal hyperplasia (CAH), polycystic ovaries and some testicular tumours.

Plasma Adrenocorticotrophin (ACTH)

Normal

9.00 a.m.	25–100 ng/l
6.00 p.m.	< 50 ng/l

ACTH levels are measured by radioimmunoassay and are only available from supraregional centres. Blood samples must be collected into heparinized plastic tubes cooled on ice, separated immediately, and the plasma frozen at $-20°C$ until assayed, since ACTH is unstable in plasma. In Cushing's syndrome a very low level confirms a primary adrenal tumour, whereas a normal or slightly raised level excludes this and suggests a pituitary lesion. A level over 1000 ng/l favours ectopic ACTH secretion. Primary adrenal failure is confirmed by a low cortisol level and a high ACTH level.

Urine Pregnanetriol

Normal

Adult males	1.2–7.5 μmol per 24 h
Adult females	
(follicular phase)	0.3–5.3 μmol per 24 h
(luteal phase)	2.7–6.5 μmol per 24 h
Infants	< 0.6 μmol per 24 h
Children (2– 5 years)	1.5 μmol per 24 h
(5–15 years)	< 4.5 μmol per 24 h

It is a metabolite of 17-OH progesterone, a cortisol precursor, and excretion is increased in pregnancy, congenital adrenal hyperplasia, polycystic ovaries, and ovarian and adrenal tumours.

Serum 17-α-Hydroxyprogesterone

Normal

Adult females	concentrations are highest in the morning and vary with the menstrual cycle. Levels rise in congenital adrenal hyperplasia, especially 21-β-hydroxylase deficiency.
Neonates	< 13 nmol/l

ADRENAL ANTIBODIES

These are found in about 50% of patients with idiopathic Addison's disease and appear early. They may occur in other autoimmune diseases.

DYNAMIC TESTS

Tetracosactrin (Synacthen) Test
Tetracosactrin plain 250 μg i.v. is given after breakfast at 9.00 a.m. and plasma cortisol levels are measured before and 30 minutes, 60 minutes and 5 hours after.

Normal

Basal level	330– 770 nmol/l
Maximum level	550–1100 nmol/l (usually at 30 min.)
Increment	220– 690 nmol/l

An impaired response is seen in primary and secondary adrenal failure. In Cushing's syndrome no response is seen with adrenal carcinoma and adenoma, but a normal or exaggerated response is seen in pituitary dependent disease. There is no set pattern with the ectopic ACTH syndrome. The test can be usefully combined with assessment of the diurnal cortisol rhythm if plasma cortisol is measured at 11.00 p.m. the previous night.

Long Tetracosactrin Test
Tetracosactrin depot 2 mg i.m. is given for three days and the standard test is repeated on the fourth day.

In secondary adrenal failure the plasma cortisol level rises above 700 nmol/l, but in primary failure it stays below 280 nmol/l after tetracosactrin. Prednisolone 5 mg twice daily may be given concurrently if adrenal crisis is feared.

Dexamethasone Suppression Tests
Dexamethasone is a powerful steroid which suppresses ACTH production, as measured by plasma and urinary steroids, but does not interfere with the usual measurements because it is present in plasma at very low concentrations.

Screening test
Dexamethasone 2 mg is taken at bedtime and the plasma cortisol should be less than 170 nmol/l on waking. High values are seen with Cushing's syndrome, but also stress, oestrogens and complicated diabetes. This test can be used for outpatient screening.

Low-dose test

Dexamethasone 0.5 mg is given six-hourly for forty-eight hours, urine is collected on the second day and plasma cortisol is measured on the morning of the third day.

Normally plasma cortisol is below 170 nmol/l and urinary cortisol is below 170 nmol per 24 h, but not in Cushing's syndrome.

High-dose test

Dexamethasone 2 mg is given six-hourly for forty-eight hours. Urinary cortisol is measured on the day before and the two days of the test. Plasma cortisol is measured with the first dose at 9.00 a.m. and with the last dose at 9.00 a.m. This test helps with the differentiation of the causes of Cushing's syndrome. In adrenal hyperplasia due to a pituitary adenoma, plasma and urinary steroids often, but not always, fall to less than 50% of the control values. In adrenal neoplasms and the ectopic ACTH syndrome there is usually no suppression. It is often convenient to run the low- and high-dose tests consecutively, with a basal day and four dexamethasone days.

Metyrapone (Metopirone) test

Metyrapone blocks the last step in cortisol synthesis, lowering the plasma cortisol level, which in turn, stimulates ACTH production. Therefore, if the adrenals are responsive to ACTH, metyrapone causes an increased production of cortisol precursors (serum 11-deoxycortisol and urinary 17-oxosteroids), but a suppression of serum cortisol levels. The test is unreliable in the assessment of Cushing's disease because of normal fluctuation in urinary output. Normally urinary cortisol precursors increase twofold and this increase is absent in adrenal carcinoma, adenoma and ectopic ACTH syndrome. The test may be used to assess the adequacy of the drug treatment of Cushing's disease.

Metyrapone 750 mg is given four-hourly for 24 hours. Urine collections are made for two days before, during, and one day after this period. Cortisol levels are checked four-hourly on the metyrapone day.

ADRENAL DISEASES

Adrenal Insufficiency

This may be chronic or present as a medical emergency. It may be due to primary adrenal disease or secondary to pituitary failure. Anorexia nervosa and renal failure enter into the differential diagnosis. Acute insufficiency must be distinguished from other causes of shock.

Preliminary tests
Suggestive findings include a low serum sodium, bicarbonate and fasting blood sugar, and a high serum potassium and blood urea. Electrolyte abnormalities are less common in secondary adrenal failure because aldosterone secretion is normal.

Diagnosis
An 11.00 p.m. and a 9.00 a.m. cortisol level are taken, followed by a short tetracosactrin test. Blood may usefully be stored for later ACTH estimation if necessary. In adrenal failure the short test will be abnormal even if the early morning cortisol level is still within normal limits. In primary adrenal disease the patient is often pigmented, the long Synacthen test is abnormal and the ACTH level is high. Secondary adrenal failure may be suspected in a patient who is not pigmented and here the long Synacthen test is normal and the ACTH level is low or normal. The most sensitive test for minor degrees of secondary adrenal failure is the insulin tolerance test (ITT, p. 114) where the cortisol level normally should rise by more than 220 nmol/l to a peak of over 550 nmol/l. If there is concern about the condition of the patient, a sample for cortisol and ACTH levels should be taken and the treatment with prednisolone 5 mg twice daily started. This will not interfere with the tetracosactrin tests.

Aetiology
Autoimmune adrenalitis is the commonest cause and adrenal antibodies and evidence of other endocrine deficiencies may be found. Tuberculosis is suggested by adrenal calcification or evidence of TB elsewhere. Secondary neoplasm, usually bronchial, and amyloidosis are rare causes. Secondary adrenal failure is usually due to suppression of the hypothalamic-pituitary-adrenal axis by corticosteroid drugs, but also occurs with pituitary disease (p. 111).

Acute Adrenal Insufficiency
This occurs when a patient with primary adrenal failure becomes salt

depleted, but most commonly when a patient previously treated with corticosteroids is subjected to stress.

A cortisol level should be taken and i.v. hydrocortisone then given. The usual tests may be done if the patient is maintained on prednisolone. Other types of shock may also respond to large doses of glucocorticoid. Recovery from suppression of the pituitary adrenal axis by steroid drugs can only be assumed if there is a normal cortisol diurnal rhythm and a normal response to tetracosactrin and insulin. It is usually simpler to cover surgery and intercurrent illness with extra hydrocortisone.

Cushing's Syndrome
This is suspected from the typical appearance of the patient and the preliminary tests, confirmed by the definitive tests. Its aetiology is then established. Once Cushing's syndrome has been confirmed further investigation of its cause and treatment are best carried out on a specialized unit.

Preliminary tests
Suggestive findings are hypokalaemic alkalosis and a high normal serum sodium, glycosuria and an abnormal glucose tolerance test, polycythaemia, eosinopenia, lymphocytopenia, neutrophil leucocytosis, and osteoporosis.

Definitive tests
Where clinical suspicion is weak it is reasonable to try to rule out the diagnosis before admission by outpatient urine cortisol estimation and an overnight dexamethasone test.

1. Cortisol levels—loss of the diurnal rhythm with a plasma cortisol above 220 nmol/l at 11.00 p.m. in the just awakened patient is very suggestive (but occasionally due to stress). Several estimations must be made as elevation can be phasic. It is the best initial inpatient test, but is delayed for twenty-four hours after admission to allow the patient to acclimatize to hospital.
2. Urine-free cortisol—this may be raised with obesity and stress and only intermittently raised in Cushing's syndrome. Several collections must be made. Persistent low normal levels provide good negative evidence.

3. Dexamethasone suppression test—this helps to determine the aetiology, as well as confirming the presence of the syndrome. The overnight test can be used on outpatients. Rarely a patient under stress requires 8 mg rather than 2 mg of dexamethasone daily for suppression.

Aetiology
Radiology of the pituitary fossa or adrenal glands may be helpful.

1. Iatrogenic—corticosteroid and ACTH administration. The commonest cause.
2. Adrenal hyperplasia (Cushing's disease)—caused by a pituitary tumour or unexplained pituitary hyperfunction. The response to tetracosactrin and metyrapone is increased. Plasma ACTH level is in the high normal range. Dexamethasone may suppress urine steroid excretion. There may be evidence of a pituitary tumour (p. 111).
3. Adrenal adenoma and carcinoma—these are less common than adrenal hyperplasia. There is no response to high-dose dexamethasone, tetracosactrin or metyrapone and ACTH levels are very low. With carcinoma, hypokalaemic alkalosis is more common and urine 17-oxosteroids may be elevated. The tumour may be identified by radiology.
4. Ectopic ACTH syndrome—the main manifestation may be hypokalaemia. Typically there is no response to tetracosactrin, metyrapone or dexamethasone, but here the ACTH level is very high. The tumour responsible is sought by chest X-ray and especially pelvic examination. Difficulty arises in rare cases where the tumour responds to stimuli like a normal pituitary gland.

Congenital Adrenal Hyperplasia (CAH)
Congenital enzyme deficiency causes abnormal steroid synthesis, with a deficiency of cortisol and sometimes of aldosterone. A low cortisol level causes ACTH stimulation and increased production of steroid precursors and abnormal metabolites which can be detected in the urine and plasma. The clinical picture depends on the particular enzyme deficiency. 21-Hydroxylase deficiency is the commonest disorder. Virilization of the female may present at any age and precocious puberty occurs in males. Some present with neonatal Addisonian crisis due to aldosterone deficiency. Urine 17-

oxosteroids and pregnanetriol excretion is increased. Plasma 17-OH progesterone levels are high from birth. All values are adjusted for age. ACTH levels are high and ACTH administration accentuates abnormal steroid excretion. Fractionation of urinary steroids into 11-oxy and 11-deoxy compounds may give further evidence about the enzyme deficiency.

ALDOSTERONE

Renin, formed in the juxtaglomerular apparatus of the kidney, activates angiotensin, which is a potent vasoconstrictor and also stimulates production of aldosterone. Aldosterone causes renal sodium retention and potassium excretion. Renin secretion is normally stimulated by extracellular fluid volume depletion, but may be pathologically increased. Aldosterone secretion is stimulated by severe hyperkalaemia, as well as renin. Primary aldosteronism (Conn's syndrome) is associated with high aldosterone and low renin levels and presents with hypertension and hypokalaemia but not oedema. Secondary aldosteronism caused by changes in intravascular pressure or volume, as in cirrhosis, nephrotic syndrome and cardiac failure, is associated with oedema. It also occurs with renal ischaemia, as in malignant hypertension, renal artery stenosis and chronic renal disease, and here hypertension, hyponatraemia and hypokalaemia may result. Diuretic drugs stimulate renin secretion.

Aldosterone deficiency causes hyperkalaemia and sodium depletion. It is usually part of Addison's disease, but can occur in isolation.

Plasma Renin
Heparinized plasma must be separated immediately. Patients should be off all drugs, especially antihypertensive agents, for three weeks. They should be on an adequate sodium intake. Samples are taken after overnight recumbency and rise after four hours' ambulation.

Serum Aldosterone
The patients should be on an adequate sodium intake. Recumbent and ambulant samples are taken.

Diagnosis of Primary Aldosteronism (Conn's Syndrome)

This condition does not account for more than 1% of hypertensives. Adenoma is commoner than hyperplasia.

1. Serum potassium.
   - (a) The diagnosis is unlikely if the serum level is persistently over 3.9 mmol/l or the plasma level is over 3.6 mmol/l in the untreated patient. The potassium level is taken without occlusion or exercise of the arm and the serum is separated quickly.
   - (b) Hypokalaemia may become severe with diuretics. The diagnosis is suspected if the serum potassium is still below 3.5 mmol/l and the urine potassium is over 40 mmol/l four days after diuretics have been stopped.
   - (c) A high sodium diet (200 mmol/day) for one week improves hypokalaemia in secondary aldosteronism by suppressing aldosterone production, but aggravates it in Conn's syndrome.
2. Serum sodium—levels are often over 140 mmol/l, whereas they are usually below 135 mmol/l in secondary aldosteronism because sodium concentration is inversely proportional to renin secretion. Intermediate levels do not exclude either diagnosis.
3. Plasma hormones—renin levels are low and aldosterone levels are high. Renin levels are not increased by ambulation or sodium depletion. Aldosterone levels are not suppressed by saline infusion.
4. Therapeutic test—spironolactone 300 mg daily controls most patients with Conn's syndrome. It will also improve hypotension or hypokalaemia of any cause, though its antihypertensive effect is more marked in Conn's syndrome than in secondary aldosteronism.
5. Radiology—a tumour may be visualized by CT.

Hypertension and Hypokalaemia

The following are considered:

1. Drugs—diuretics, corticosteroids, carbenoxolone, liquorice.
2. Secondary aldosteronism (p. 107).
3. Two separate diseases.
4. Adrenal disease—primary aldosteronism, phaeochromocytoma and Cushing's syndrome.

ADRENAL MEDULLA

The catecholamine hormones adrenaline and noradrenaline break down to metadrenaline and normetadrenaline and then both to vanillylmandelic acid (VMA). Dopamine, the precursor of the hormones, breaks down to homovanillic acid (HVA). Catecholamine hormone secretion is assessed by measuring urinary excretion of the hormones and their metabolites. Excessive secretion occurs with phaeochromocytoma, neuroblastoma and ganglioneuroma.

Urine tests
To avoid false-positives and false-negatives it is best that no drugs, caffeine, chocolate, vanilla products or bananas are taken for four days before urine collection. Methyldopa does not affect VMA excretion but beta-blocking drugs can affect many assays. The laboratory must be informed of any drug being taken. Spectrophotometric methods are less subject to drug interference than fluorimetry. Samples should be collected into 10 ml hydrochloric acid and refrigerated.

Urine Total Metadrenalines (Metanephrines, Methylated Amines)

Normal
Adults

0.5–7.0 μmol per 24 h; 0.03–0.69 mmol metanephrine per mol creatinine.
An excretion of below 7.0 μmol per 24 h is good evidence against a tumour and a level of over 15 μmol per 24 h is very suggestive.

Infants

0.2–1.7 mmol per mol creatinine falling gradually in children to adult levels.

Urine Vanillylmandelic Acid (VMA)

Normal

Adults	10–35 μmol per 24 h
Neonates	0– 5 μmol per 24 h
Infants	0–10 μmol per 24 h
Children	5–25 μmol per 24 h or 0.9–4 mmol per mol creatinine

This is the easiest substance to measure and present in the largest amount. It is the best screening test and is especially useful in the diagnosis of neuroblastoma.

Homovanillic Acid (HVA)

Normal
Adults   < 82 μmol per 24 h
Children   1.9–10.0 mmol per mol creatinine

Increased excretion is commoner with malignant phaeochromocytoma and neuroblastoma.

Diagnosis of Phaeochromocytoma

This should be considered where hypertension is associated with suggestive features and in any severe hypertension. Impaired glucose tolerance, mild hypokalaemia, a riased haematocrit and a low plasma volume may occur. Positive urine tests are necessary for diagnosis. VMA and one other measurement should always be made. Phenolic acid chromatography is one qualitative screening method which picks up HVA and VMA. Two negative results almost exclude a tumour. The tumour is located by i.v. urography, computerized tomography or angiography. It may arise in the adrenal gland or elsewhere in the neural crest.

Chapter Eleven

DISEASES OF THE PITUITARY AND GONADS

ANTERIOR PITUITARY

Releasing and release-inhibiting hormones of the hypothalamus control pituitary production of trophic hormones which stimulate the target endocrine glands to produce their secretions. These in turn feed back to reduce hypothalamic or pituitary activity. The anterior pituitary hormones are growth hormone (GH), prolactin, follicle-stimulating hormone (FSH), luteinizing hormone (LH), corticotrophin (ACTH) and thyrotrophin (TSH). Most are measured by radioimmunoassay (RIA). Hypothalamic hormones appear to control the release of ACTH, GH, TSH, LH and FSH. Thyrotrophin-releasing hormone (TRH) and gonadotrophin-releasing hormone (LH/FSH-RH) are in clinical use.

Hypothalamic and Pituitary Disease
This may present with evidence of a space-occupying lesion, hypopituitarism or of increased secretion of a hormone by a functioning adenoma.

Space-occupying lesions present with pituitary dysfunction, headache and visual disturbance, especially changes in the visual fields, and are confirmed radiologically by skull X-ray and tomography. Functioning adenomas usually secrete GH, prolactin, or ACTH in excess. Pituitary failure is caused by tumours arising from or near the pituitary by infiltrations or infarction. Failure of gonadotrophin and GH secretion usually precedes failure of other trophic hormones and they are the commonest two deficiencies to occur in isolation.

Pituitary Function Tests
The first step is to measure basal pituitary and target hormone levels.

111

The target gland hormones are cortisol, oestrogens, progesterone, thyroxine (T4) and tri-iodothyronine (T3), and the pituitary hormones are GH, LH, FSH, ACTH, TSH and prolactin, as above.

In primary target-organ failure, reduced target hormone levels are associated with raised pituitary hormone levels, e.g. low T4 and high TSH. With pituitary or hypothalamic failure, target and pituitary hormone levels are low. Tests stimulating the hypothalamus, e.g. insulin hypoglycaemia test, or the pituitary, e.g. TRH test, are necessary. Pituitary hyperfunction is usually associated with hyper-prolactinaemia or raised growth hormone levels.

Growth Hormone (GH)

Normal
Clotted blood in fasting state, preferably from an indwelling needle.

Adult males	$< 2 \mu g/l$
Adult females	$< 10 \mu g/l$
Children	$0–20 \mu g/l$
Elderly males	$0–10 \mu g/l$
Elderly females	$1–14 \mu g/l$

Production is phasic. Suspected hypofunction must be checked by a stimulation test, and hyperfunction by a glucose load.

Suppression test
This is used in the investigation of gigantism and acromegaly. A standard glucose tolerance test is performed and GH levels will normally be suppressed below 1.5 $\mu g/l$ at 1½ to 3 hours after the glucose load.

Stimulation tests
These are used in the investigation of growth failure. The GH level should reach 10 $\mu g/l$. A positive response in the exercise or Bovril test obviates the need for other tests, but a negative response must be checked by insulin hypoglycaemia.
1. Bovril test—Bovril 30 g per 1.5 sq m body surface is given in warm water and half-hourly samples are taken for two hours.
2. Exercise test—GH is measured twenty minutes after ten minutes vigorous exercise.

3. Glucagon test—GH is measured hourly for three hours after glucagon 1 mg s.c. or i.m.
4. Insulin tolerance test (ITT)—this is the definitive test.

Prolactin

Normal
Elevation occurs with stress and samples are best taken from an indwelling needle. Moderate rises should be rechecked.

Adult males   < 20 μg/l
Adult females
 (follicular phase)   < 23 μg/l, (luteal phase) 5–40 μg/l

Deficiency causes failure of lactation and is always associated with failure of other hormones. Increase can cause varying combinations of gynaecomastia, galactorrhoea, infertility, secondary amenorrhoea, dysfunctional uterine bleeding and impotence. It interferes with the effects of gonadotrophins on the gonads and inhibits gonadotrophin release.

Increase
1. Pituitary and hypothalamic disease – adenomas, functional hypersecretion.
2. Drugs – oestrogens, TRH, methyldopa, reserpine, phenothiazines, haloperidol, metoclopramide, cimetidine.
3. Miscellaneous – renal failure, hypothyroidism, chest wall disease

Gonadotrophins
Hypothalamic LH/FSH-RH stimulates pituitary FSH and LH release. FSH stimulates spermatogenesis in the male and oestrogen secretion in the female. LH induces ovulation and stimulates the interstitial cells of the testes. The target hormones switch off gonadotrophin production. Gonadotrophin deficiency causes delayed puberty, with near normal growth if GH secretion is normal, and after puberty loss of secondary sex characteristics, with infertility and amenorrhoea. Isolated measurements are of limited value. In primary hypogonadism, oestrogen or testosterone levels are low, gonadotrophin levels are high, there is an increased gonadotrophin response to LH/FSH-RH, and no response to clomiphene. In

pituitary failure, gonadotrophin levels are low and there is a reduced response to LH/FSH-RH and clomiphene.

Serum Follicle-Stimulating Hormone (FSH)

Adult males	1– 6 IU/l
Adult females	1– 9 IU/l, (midcycle peak < 30 IU/l)
Postmenopausal females	30–100 IU/l
Before puberty	0– 3.5 IU/l

Serum Luteinizing Hormone (LH)

Adult males	2– 9 IU/l
Adult females	2–15 IU/l (midcycle peak 30–60 IU/l)
Postmenopausal females	23–70 IU/l
Before puberty	0– 3.5 IU/l

Stimulation Tests

1. Gondadotrophin-releasing hormone (LH/FSH/RH) test—after vein cannulation, basal LH and FSH levels are taken and LH/FSH-RH 100 μg i.v. is given. LH and FSH levels are taken at 20 minutes and 60 minutes. Prior hormone treatment is best avoided as its effects on the test are variable. FSH should rise by 50% or by more than 1.5 IU/l. LH rises to five times the basal level or by 10–50 IU/l.
2. Clomiphene Test—Clomiphene 50–100 mg is given daily for ten days. LH and FSH levels are measured before and on the 4th, 7th and 10th days, and should rise above normal. Clomiphene blocks the inhibitory effect of gonadal steroids on the hypothalamus, causing a rise in FSH and LH. This rise is absent in hypothalamic and pituitary disease and anorexia nervosa.

Insulin Tolerance Test (ITT)

After preliminary measurement of basal hormones (p. 112) an ITT is a sensitive test for pituitary failure or hypothalamic dysfunction. The test is precluded by epilepsy, myocardial ischaemia, or a morning cortisol level below 165 nmol/l. Intravenous 50% dextrose and hydrocortisone must be available. Adequate hypoglycaemia with a blood glucose below 2.2 mmol/l must be produced and a repeat insulin dose may be given at 45 minutes if it is not, as judged by the absence of sweating and a blood glucose measurement. The insulin dose is 0.10 U/kg, but 0.15 U/kg in the obese and up to 0.3 U/kg in untreated acromegaly or Cushing's disease.

Method
1. 8.30 a.m.—vein cannulation of the fasting, resting patient with a heparinized butterfly needle.
2. 9.00 a.m.—basal GH, cortisol, prolactin, and blood glucose. Soluble insulin i.v. washed into vein.
3. Repeat estimations at 9.30, 9.45, 10.00, 10.30 and 11.00 a.m. Finish with i.v. dextrose.

Normal result
Cortisol rises by 200 nmol/l to 500 nmol/l, GH reaches 10 µg/l (20 mu/l), and prolactin reaches 25 µg/l (800 mu/l).

Outpatient Pituitary Function Test
1. Measure basal hormone concentrations.
2. Give TRH 100 µg + LH/FSH-RH 100 µg and tetracosactrin (p. 102) 250 µg i.v.
3. At 30 minutes measure TSH and prolactin (stimulated by TRH), LH and FSH (stimulated by LH/FSH-RH) and cortisol and GH (stimulated by tetracosactrin, although GH does not always respond).

POSTERIOR PITUITARY

The posterior pituitary secretes oxytocin and vasopressin (ADH) initially synthesized in the hypothalamus. Vasopressin controls renal water excretion and its secretion is stimulated primarily by an increase in plasma osmolality but also by a fall in blood volume. Deficiency causes polyuria (p. 234).

TESTES

The testes secrete testosterone and produce spermatozoa under pituitary control. Abnormality results in failure of secondary sexual development and infertility. Investigation may involve measurement of androgens, gonadotrophins, semen analysis, chromosome analysis and X-rays of the skull and hands (p. 111). Testosterone in females comes mainly from the adrenals. An excess may occur in some conditions which cause virilization.

Serum Testosterone

Normal

Adult males	11–36 nmol/l
Adult females	1–3.0 nmol/l
Prepubertal	< 0.5 nmol/l

Plasma 17-OH androgens can also be measured, but this is less specific.

Semen Analysis
The volume is normally 2.5–6 ml, the sperm count is 20–60 × 10^6/ml and 60% of spermatozoa should be motile and normal.

OVARY

The ovary produces oestrogens which are responsible for endometrial proliferation and secondary sexual characteristics. Oestrone and oestradiol are the main urinary oestrogens. Oestrogens are also produced by the placenta, adrenals and testes. Progesterone is secreted by the corpus luteum after ovulation and also by the placenta and adrenals. It prepares the endometrium for implantation. Pregnanediol is an important metabolite. Secretion of both hormones is higher in the luteal than the follicular phase of the menstrual cycle and there is a periovulatory secretion peak. Androgens are also secreted and an excess produced in carcinoma or polycystic disease may cause hirsutism or amenorrhoea.

Urine Total Oestrogen

Normal
These are measured in an early morning urine sample and expressed as μmol oestrogen per mol creatinine.

Adult females
   (follicular phase)   1.5– 4.0 μmol per mol creatinine

(luteal phase)	4.0–10.0 μmol per mol creatinine
(midcycle)	6.0–20.0 μmol per mol creatinine
Pregnancy (30 weeks)	> 4 mmol per mol creatinine
(35 weeks)	> 6 mmol per mol creatinine
(40 weeks)	> 8 mmol per mol creatinine

Increased excretion, measured fluorimetrically, may be seen in gonadal tumours and Cushing's syndrome. Reduced excretion occurs in amenorrhoea, hypopituitarism and polycystic ovaries.

In pregnancy, serial measurement of urine oestrogen creatinine ratios are used in the assessment of progress and to determine the optimal time for induction of labour in conditions such as toxaemia.

Serum Oestradiol 17-β

Normal

Adult males	<300 μmol/l
Adult females	
(follicular phase)	180–1500 μmol/l
(luteal phase)	440– 800 μmol/l
(postmenopausal)	<200μmol/l

Urine Pregnanediol

Normal

Adult females	
(follicular phase)	0–8 μmol per 24 h
(luteal phase)	8–33 μmol per 24 h

High values are seen in congenital adrenal hyperplasia and low values occur in the luteal phase, when infertility is due to luteal insufficiency. Serum progesterone can also be measured.

CLINICAL PROBLEMS

Acromegaly

The disease is usually considered because of the facial appearance. Clinical evidence of increased growth of skin, viscera and bones is present. Gigantism occurs if the disease starts before epiphyseal fusion. There may be evidence of an intracranial space-occupying lesion and hypopituitarism (p. 111) also. A heel pad over 22 mm on X-ray is evidence of increased soft-tissue thickness. Impaired glucose tolerance occurs in 50% of patients. Proof is by demonstration of high growth hormone levels not adequately supressed by an oral GTT.

Delayed Growth and Puberty
Puberty usually starts in males before the age of 14 years and in females before 13 years. Scrotal rugosity is the first sign of puberty in males and breast development in females, followed by pubic hair in both. Once started, changes usually proceed normally. Delay in puberty may be associated with delay in growth. Also, short stature may become even more evident at puberty when peers experience a growth spurt. The two conditions are therefore discussed together.

Investigation is undertaken if height, radiological bone age or sexual maturation are markedly abnormal as judged by the charts available for these parameters and if there is no progress with time.

Causes
1. Familial—normal puberty may not occur until 18 years and a family history of such delay is very helpful. There are no other abnormalities. A normal response to gonadotrophin suggests puberty is imminent. Short stature also may be familial.
2. Systemic disease—usually obvious but sometimes not, e.g. coeliac disease.
3. Low birth weight—children who are 'small for dates' may remain so.
4. Social—deprivation whether nutritional or emotional.
5. Endocrine—hypothyrodism; pituitary disease including isolated growth hormone or gonadotrophin deficiency; primary hypogonadism, in which height may be normal, gonadotrophin levels are high, and chromosome studies may be abnormal; corticosteroid administration, hyperprolactinaemia. Evidence of endocrine dysfunction should be sought, as indicated elsewhere.
6. Chromosomal disorders—achondroplasia; Turner's syndrome (short females); Klinefelter's syndrome (abnormal males).

Amenorrhoea
Primary amenorrhoea should be investigated as for delayed puberty, noting that menstruation usually follows breast development. If growth and secondary sexual characteristics are normal, a pelvic abnormality is possible. The two obvious causes of secondary

amenorrhoea are pregnancy and the menopause, the latter being confirmed by low oestrogen and high FSH levels. Amenorrhoea after contraceptive pill withdrawal must be investigated if it persists. Emotional hypothalamic amenorrhoea is common but difficult to prove. Anorexia nervosa and even rapid weight gain may be responsible. Examination should exclude severe systemic disease.

Endocrine causes include:–

1. Thyroid disease (FSH high).
2. Adrenal disease—Addison's disease, Cushing's syndrome, congenital adrenal hyperplasia (FSH high).
3. Ovarian disease—Premature ovarian failure and masculinizing ovarian pathology (FSH high).
4. Pituitary disease (FSH low or normal).
5. Hyperprolactinaemia (FSH) low or normal).

A high FSH level excludes pituitary and hypothalamic disease. Withdrawal bleeding within seven days of a five-day course of medroxyprogesterone acetate 10 mg daily indicates that the uterus is normal and oestrogen secretion is normal. In oestrogen deficiency bleeding will occur if ethinyloestradiol 100 μg daily is given for 21 days and progesterone for the last five days. The various endocrine conditions are investigated, as indicated elsewhere.

Hirsutism
A definite endocrine disorder should be particularly sought if there is other evidence of virilization, amenorrhoea, or if it presents not, as usual, between the ages of 16 and 21 years, but at puberty or in early middle age.

Causes
1. Constitutional—racial, menopausal, familial and idiopathic. These are the commonest.
2. Drugs—phenytoin, corticosteroids, androgens, progestogens, diazoxide, minoxidil.
3. Ovaries—tumours, polycystic disease.
4. Adrenals—Cushing's syndrome, especially due to carcinoma, congenital adrenal hyperplasia (p. 106).

Evidence of ovarian or adrenal disease should be sought by measuring plasma testosterone, urinary 17-oxosteroids and 17-hydroxysteroids, urinary pregnanediol and pregnanetriol, and plasma 17-hydroxyprogesterone levels. Laparoscopy and computerized tomography may be necessary to define adrenal or ovarian pathology.

Chapter Twelve

DIABETES MELLITUS AND HYPOGLYCAEMIA

DIABETES MELLITUS

Diabetes mellitus is a disease state associated with the production of insufficient insulin to achieve normal metabolism and in the diabetic state abnormal carbohydrate, fat and protein metabolism occur. Diabetes mellitus is assessed clinically by measuring changes in glucose and fat metabolism as shown by tests on urine and blood. When dipstick and tablet tests are used, the maker's instructions must be followed exactly.

Urine Glucose

Normal
Less than 1 mmol/l. Dipsticks and tablet tests are negative. Glucose usually appears in the urine when the blood glucose exceeds the average renal threshold level of 10 mmol/l. The threshold may be low especially in the young and glycosuria does not always imply hyperglycaemia (p. 122). In the elderly and when the glomerular filtration rate is reduced, the renal threshold may be high and hyperglycaemia may be present without glycosuria. The glucose concentration of the urine may lag behind that of the blood, especially if it has been in the bladder for some time. It is also an insensitive guide to the blood glucose level, as the urine will be negative if the blood glucose is between 0 and 10 mmol/l. The urine of infants must be screened by Clinitest (Ames) as stick tests detect only glucose and not other sugars.

Tablet tests
Clinitest is a copper reduction method and can measure glycosuria from 10–110 mmol/l (0.2–2.0%). If two drops of urine instead of five are used, it is semiquantitative up to 5% (280 mmol/l). It is positive with some other sugars and false-positives occur with drugs such as Vitamin C, salicylates and some antibiotics.

Dipstick tests
These (e.g. Clinistix, Ames) rely on glucose oxidase and are sensitive and specific for glucose. False-negatives can occur in the presence of ketones, so they are unreliable with ketosis prone insulin-dependent diabetes. Occasional false-negatives occur with aspirin and Vitamin C, which latter may be incorporated in tetracycline tablets. False-positives occur when the urine container is contaminated by detergents. The sticks must be fresh and the correct technique used.

Several stick tests are available. They detect glucose down to a concentration of 5 mmol/l and are the most convenient way of excluding glycosuria. In quantitative terms they are less reliable than Clinitest and therefore less suitable for controlling diabetes.

Glycosuria Without Diabetes

With transient hyperglycaemia
1. Acute intracranial disease, e.g. cerebral haemorrhage.
2. Lag storage curve (alimentary oxyhyperglycaemia, thyrotoxicosis).
3. Stress, e.g. myocardial infarction. This may also cause exacerbation of a genuine mild diabetic state.

Without hyperglycaemia
1. Pregnancy—it commonly occurs, especially in the second half, due to a rise in the glomerular filtration rate.
2. Renal glycosuria—a not uncommon isolated and partial functional defect of glucose reabsorption in the proximal tubules is seen most often in younger people.
3. Proximal tubular disease (p. 232).
4. Renal failure.
5. Heavy proteinuria.

Plasma Glucose

Normal (fasting)
Whole blood in fluoride tube

Adults	3.5–6.0 mmol/l
Neonates	1.7–4.4 mmol/l
Premature infants	1.1–3.3 mmol/l
Children	3.3–5.5 mmol/l

Measurement can be by the reducing properties of glucose or by glucose oxidase. Modern reducing methods, e.g. the automated ferricyanide method, record only slightly higher values than glucose oxidase methods. Serum and plasma levels are about 10% above whole blood, depending on the haematocrit.

Fluoridated plasma samples are stable for 8 hours at room temperature and 3 days if refrigerated.

Glucose levels are similar in capillary and venous blood in the normal fasting state, but after food and in hyperglycaemic states capillary levels may be over 2 mmol/l higher and this is relevant with glucose tolerance tests.

Rapid tests
These tests utilize paper strips and capillary blood from a finger prick. They usefully provide rapid confirmation of the presence of hypoglycaemia or hyperglycaemia. The correct technique must be carefully followed and measurements should be confirmed by samples sent to the laboratory, as they are semiquantitative. The strips are read by eye but accuracy can be improved with a small meter and the method can then be used to achieve a tight control of diabetes. Dextrostix (Ames) and BM-Test Glycemie 20–800 (Boehringer) are available.

Effect of Changes in Blood Glucose Concentration
Hyperglycaemia stimulates insulin and suppresses growth hormone production, though not always in the diabetic. It may cause glycosuria and renal loss of water and electrolytes. Hypoglycaemia stimulates the production of those pituitary hormones stimulated by stress and suppresses insulin release. It may present with coma, convulsions or episodic abnormal behaviour. Sometimes very low glucose levels are tolerated without symptoms. The classical sweating and tachycardia do not always occur.

Oral Glucose Tolerance Test (OGTT)

A standard oral glucose tolerance test (OGTT) is necessary only if the diagnosis is not confirmed or refuted by the simpler tests below. It should be carried out before dietary treatment, as carbohydrate restriction impairs tolerance, although weight loss ultimately improves it. It is done in the morning after an overnight fast and the patient must rest and not smoke during the test. Adults are given 75 g of glucose in 100–200 ml of chilled flavoured water and children are given 1.75 g/kg to a maximum of 50 g. Blood and urine samples are taken hourly or half-hourly for glucose estimation.

Diagnosis of Diabetes Mellitus

1. With classical symptoms and glycosuria—a fasting venous plasma glucose level of 8 mmol/l or more is diagnostic. If the fasting concentration is 6.8 mmol/l, a 75 g oral glucose load is given, and a two-hour venous plasma glucose level of over 11 mmol/l confirms diabetes. A two-hour level of 8–11 mmol/l is regarded as impaired glucose tolerance. Such patients are at risk of large vessel disease, but not microangiopathy.
2. Without symptoms—at least two abnormal plasma glucose values are required, e.g. a fasting level of over 8 mmol/l and a two-hour post-glucose level of over 11 mmol/l or two post-glucose levels of over 11 mmol/l (one-hour and two-hour).
3. Exclusion of diabetes mellitus
   (a) A fasting blood glucose level of below 6 mmol/l.
   (b) A blood glucose level of below 6 mmol/l two hours after a 75 g oral glucose load given at any time.

Non-diabetic Abnormalities of the Glucose Tolerance Test

Oxyhyperglycaemic curve (lag storage)

The peak level is high but the two-hour level is normal or low. This is seen especially after gastric operations and with duodenal ulcer (alimentary hyperglycaemia), but it is also seen with hyperthyroidism, liver disease and sometimes in normals.

Flat curve

The peak level is less than 1.5 mmol/l above the fasting level. This occurs with malabsorption, insulinomas, Addison's disease and hypopituitarism, but it is not unusual in normals, especially if exercise is taken during the test.

Exaggerated hypoglycaemic phase
If measurement is continued for five hours, the glucose level commonly drops to 1 mmol/l below the fasting level at one point. In some patients it drops to definite hypoglycaemic levels within three hours, but even this is only significant if there are associated hypoglycaemic symptoms. Symptomatic reactive hypoglycaemia is classically seen after gastrectomy, in association with oxyhyperglycaemia ('dumping syndrome'), and is caused by rapid absorption of carbohydrate from the jejunum and an exaggerated insulin response. It also occurs with insulinoma, rarely as an early manifestation of diabetes, and sometimes purely as a functional syndrome.

Secondary Causes of Impaired Glucose Tolerance
1. Pancreatic disease—acute and chronic pancreatitis and haemochromatosis.
2. Endocrine hyperfunction—Cushing's syndrome (cortisol), phaeochromocytoma (adrenaline), acromegaly (growth hormone), primary aldosteronism (hypokalaemia).
3. Drug induced—thiazide diuretics slightly aggravate existing diabetes, partly through hypokalaemia, but with the exception of diazoxide, do not usually affect normal subjects. Corticosteroids markedly impair and oestrogens, including the contraceptive pill, may slightly impair glucose tolerance. Poisoning by salicylates, Epanutin or carbon monoxide may cause hyperglycaemia.
4. Miscellaneous—renal failure, liver failure, malignancy and stress such as myocardial infarction or emotion. Pre-existing diabetes may become clinically manifest.
5. Pregnancy—glycosuria is usually renal. Pregnancy aggravates existing diabetes but may cause slight impairment of glucose tolerance in normals. The situation is carefully monitored and the OGTT is repeated six weeks after delivery in doubtful cases.

Assessment of Diabetic Control
The urine glucose and blood glucose measured in the clinic give no indication of control during the previous weeks. The record of the urine tests carried out at home is dependent on the reliability of the patient. The urine test should be negative after the main meal.

Reliable patients can measure their own blood glucose using a finger prick and a stick test, preferably with a glucose meter. The fasting level should be below 6.5 mmol/l and the post-prandial level below 8 mmol/l. A further advance has been the measurement of glycosylated haemoglobin (GHb), which is not dependent on patient co-operation.

The degree of control which can be expected depends on the age and circumstances of the patient.

Glycosylated Haemoglobin (GHb)

When the haemoglobin molecule is exposed to glucose its beta-chain irreversibly acquires glucose molecules. Normally 3–6% of haemoglobin is glycosylated (HbA_{1C}). This figure may rise to 20% in uncontrolled diabetes. The HbA_{1C} level reflects average blood glucose levels in the previous month. An excess of young red cells, as in haemolytic anaemia, gives falsely low results.

Ketosis

When glucose cannot be adequately metabolized, the metabolism of fat results in ketoacidosis. An excess of hydrogen ions and ketone bodies, acetoacetate, β-hydroxybutyrate and acetone are produced. Ketosis assumes especial importance in diabetes mellitus, but it is also seen with vomiting, starvation, dehydration, alcoholism and salicylate poisoning. It tends to occur easily in pregnancy and childhood.

Urine Ketones

Normally none are detectable, but when ketosis occurs they are found in the urine before the plasma becomes positive. The usual tests are very sensitive and one should confirm that ketosis is severe by demonstrating a positive test in the plasma or by the ferric chloride test. Acetest (Ames) is a tablet test and there is also a dipstick test, both containing nitroprusside. They are especially specific for acetoacetate and do not pick up β-hydroxybutyrate. Both are very sensitive and trace reactions in diabetes may be just related to fasting. False-positives occur with phthalein compounds and laevodopa and false-negatives occur with stale urine or outdated reagents.

Ferric chloride test (Gerhardt)
Ferric chloride 10% is added dropwise to urine and a deep red colour develops if the urine acetoacetate concentration is above about 50 mg per 100 ml. Salicylates give a false-positive, but Acetest is negative or weakly positive in this case.

Serum Ketones
These are measured on serial dilutions of serum with Acetest as for urine and are a guide to the severity of ketosis. The serum is always positive in significant ketosis.

Diagnosis of Diabetic Coma
In hypoglycaemic coma a blood sugar should always be taken before glucose is given. In hyperglycaemic coma or precoma there is usually heavy glycosuria and ketonuria, though exceptions do occur.
1. No glycosuria—this may occur when there is associated severe oliguric renal failure or severe acidosis.
2. No ketonuria
   (a) In severe renal failure ketonaemia occurs without ketonuria.
   (b) Hyperosmolar coma—blood sugar and sometimes serum sodium levels are very high. Acidosis may be absent. It occurs particularly in dehydrated elderly patients and when thirst is relieved by sweet drinks.
   (c) Lactic acidosis—there is hyperglycaemia and acidosis but no ketonaemia. Often this is associated with phenformin treatment or Gram-negative septicaemia.

HYPOGLYCAEMIA

Diagnosis requires the presence of symptoms (p. 123) with a blood sugar below 2.2 mmol/l and relief of symptoms by i.v. glucose. Apart from reactive hypoglycaemia, it is related to fasting. If suspected, blood must be taken for glucose and insulin estimation, if appropriate, before glucose is given.

Causes
1. Reactive hypoglycaemia—this is seen in the conditions associated with an oxyhyperglycaemic curve (p. 124) and is diagnosed by an extended glucose tolerance test.

2. Endocrine failure—hypopituitarism, hypoadrenalism, myxoedema coma.
3. Hepatic failure—poisoning, hepatitis.
4. Insulinoma.
5. Neoplasms—especially large retroperitoneal sarcomas.
6. Drug induced.
   (a) Usually insulin overdose, but also sulphonylureas, especially a long-acting drug like chlorpropamide in elderly people with renal impairment.
   (b) Alcohol—excessive amounts in diabetes, in adolescents trying it out, and in malnourished alcoholics.
   (c) Poisoning by carbon tetrachloride, paracetamol or aspirin (paracetamol causes falsely high blood glucose levels with some methods of measurement).
7. Paediatric—infants of diabetic mothers, immature infants, leucine or fructose intolerance, glycogen storage disease, galactosaemia, and sometimes reactive hypoglycaemia.

Plasma Insulin

Normal
Heparinized blood after a 15-hour fast. Plasma must be separated immediately and frozen.

3–13 mIU/l (at normal fasting blood glucose concentrations)

It is measured by a radioimmunoassay which also measures to some extent biologically inactive insulin precursors and cannot be used in subjects who have received insulin because of the presence of antibodies. In a normal subject a plasma glucose level of below 2 mmol/l is associated with a plasma insulin level of below 1.5 mIU/l. A plasma insulin level of above 5 mIU/l in the presence of symptomatic hypoglycaemia is inappropriately high and suggestive of an insulinoma, but may also be found with islet cell hyperplasia, insulin and sulphonylurea administration and after gastrectomy. Measurement is useful only in the differential diagnosis of spontaneous hypoglycaemia.

Diagnosis of Insulinoma
Hypoglycaemic symptoms occurring with fasting or exertion in an otherwise healthy adult suggest a pancreatic beta-cell tumour. When suspicision arises, symptomatic fasting hypoglycaemia with

inappropriate insulin secretion should be demonstrated on at least two occasions. Normally, spontaneous hypoglycaemia occurs, but it may be useful to fast the patient from 10.00 p.m. and prolong the fast until hypoglycaemia occurs, often at 6.00 a.m. but sometimes not until 12 noon or later. Close observation and two-hourly blood glucose measurements are necessary. If the fast is extended beyond 24 hours, normal lean females may become hypoglycaemic. The typical syndrome will usually occur:

1. Blood sugar level below 2.2 mmol/l.
2. Appropriate symptoms relieved by glucose.
3. Inappropriately high insulin level.

Provocative tests

Continued production of endogenous insulin by an insulinoma during hypoglycaemia can be demonstrated if hypoglycaemia is induced by fish insulin. Alternatively, beef or pork insulin may be used and the plasma concentration of the species-specific C-peptide associated with insulin can be determined.

An insulinoma will also show an exaggerated secretion of insulin in response to tolbutamide.

Tolbutamide test

This somewhat dangerous test is used mainly to exclude an insulinoma when prolonged fasting does not produce hypoglycaemia. Dextrose 50% and hydrocortisone are available and the preliminary blood glucose is normal. Tolbutamide 1 g i.v. is given through a cannula to the fasting patient and blood is taken for glucose and insulin before and at 5, 10, 15, 30, 60, 120 and 180 minutes. Normally, the blood glucose level falls by 50% and returns to 70% of the fasting level at 180 mins. With insulinomas, the blood glucose level falls further and does not recover. The plasma insulin level in one of the first four samples rises to over 120 mIU/l.

In other forms of hypoglycaemia the insulin response is usually normal.

Localization

Coeliac axis and superior mesenteric artery angiography are carried out, but often fail to locate the tumour before surgery. Measurement of gastrin, glucagon and vasoactive polypeptide levels may help to determine the nature of the hyperfunctioning tissue.

Chapter Thirteen

METABOLIC DISEASE

LIPIDS

Lipids are insoluble in water and occur in the blood as complexes with apoproteins. Measurement of serum triglyceride and cholesterol is sufficient for the management of most patients with hyperlipidaemia. Full classification of a hyperlipidaemia requires measurement of the cholesterol content of high-density lipoprotein (HDL-cholesterol) and chylomicron estimation also. Visual examination of refrigerated serum is also useful. Fredrickson classifies hyperlipidaemias by lipoprotein electrophoresis.

Lipids should be measured after a 15-hour fast without venous stasis and with the patient seated for 15 minutes. The patient should be well and taking his usual food and alcohol intake. Severe illness lowers cholesterol and raises triglyceride concentrations for a few months and minor illnesses cause transient misleading changes. The 'normal' range varies with age, sex, race, class, country, physical activity and diet. What is 'normal' is not necessarily optimal in cardiovascular terms. High carbohydrate intake and prolonged high fat intake raises triglyceride and very low-density lipoprotein levels (VLDL). Cholesterol raises the cholesterol content of low-density lipoprotein. Alcohol raises triglyceride levels and very low-density lipoprotein. Low-density lipoprotein (LDL) cholesterol promotes and high-density lipoprotein (HDL) cholesterol reduces atherosclerosis.

Serum Cholesterol

Normal
Preferably fasting. There is a small rise after food.

Adults	3.8– 7.7 mmol/l
Neonates	2.4– 5.6 mmol/l
Infants	3.1– 5.7 mmol/l
Children	3.1– 6.2 mmol/l
Elderly males	4.1– 8.9 mmol/l
Elderly females	4.7–11.2 mmol/l
Pregnancy	slight rise

Increase (hypercholesterolaemia)
1. Diabetes mellitus.
2. Hypothyroidism.
3. Nephrotic syndrome.
4. Hepatobiliary disease—especially cholestasis.
5. Primary familial (see below).
6. Drugs—alcohol, oestrogens.

Decrease (hypocholesterolaemia)
1. Malnutrition.
2. Malabsorption.
3. Severe liver disease.
4. Severe anaemias.
5. Thyrotoxicosis.
6. Inborn metabolic errors.
7. Stress—measurements are unreliable for three months after myocardial infarction or surgery and for a few days after minor illness.

Serum Triglycerides

Normal
Adult males	0.5–1.8 mmol/l
Adult females	0.5–1.6 mmol/l
Neonates	0.1–0.5 mmol/l
Infants	0.2–2.1 mmol/l
Pregnancy	0.5–2.3 mmol/l.

In general, triglyceride levels rise in the same disorders that cause hypercholesterolaemia, but hypertriglyceridaemia is particularly common in alcoholism and also occurs in renal failure and pancreatitis. Low levels occur in congenital lipoprotein deficiencies.

Serum Appearance

After 12 hours refrigeration, uniformly turbid serum indicates a high VLDL content. Clear serum with a creamy top indicates an increased chylomicron concentration. Turbid serum with a creamy top indicates VLDL and chylomicron increase.

Analysis of Lipid Abnormalities

Measurement of fasting serum cholesterol and triglyceride is sufficient for all secondary and most primary hyperlipoproteinaemias. Treatment is decided according to whether cholesterol alone or both cholesterol and triglyceride levels are raised. Primary hyperlipoproteinaemias can be classified by lipoprotein electrophoresis or ultracentrifugation (Table 13.1).

Table 13.1 Lipoprotein composition

Lipoprotein	Electrophoretic mobility	Triglyceride (%)	Cholesterol (%)
Chylomicrons	Stay at origin	90	5
Very low-density	Pre-β	70	15
Low-density	β	10	50
High-density	α₁	0	20

Phospholipid and protein content is not shown.

Fredrickson Classification

Type I — Triglyceride + + +; Cholesterol N/+; serum clear with cream top; pre-β-lipoprotein (VLDL) +. Rare, associated with pancreatitis, not vascular disease.

Type IIa — Triglyceride N; cholesterol + +; serum clear; pre-β-lipoprotein (VLDL) + +; β-lipoprotein (LDL) + +. Common, autosomal dominant, associated with vascular disease.

Type IIb — Triglyceride +; cholesterol + +; serum turbid; pre-β-lipoprotein (VLDL) +; β-lipoprotein (LDL) + +. Common, associated with vascular disease.

Type III — Triglyceride + +; cholesterol + +; serum turbid

merged pre-β- and β-lipoprotein bands (VLDL & LDL). Rare, associated with vascular disease, hyperuricaemia, abnormal glucose tolerance.

Type IV   Triglyceride +++; cholesterol N/+; serum turbid; pre-β-lipoprotein (VLDL) +++; β-lipoprotein (LDL) N/+. Very common, associated with vascular disease, abnormal glucose tolerance and hyperuricaemia.

Type V   Triglyceride +++; cholesterol ++; serum turbid + cream top; pre-β-lipoprotein (VLDL) ++; chylomicrons ++. Rare, associated with pancreatitis, abnormal glucose tolerance and hyperuricaemia, but not vascular disease.

Note that concentrations are graded N–+++. Lipid infiltration of the skin occurs with all hyperlipidaemias.

PORPHYRIAS

The porphyrias are conditions in which haem synthesis is abnormal and precursors accumulate. In acquired porphyria and congenital hepatic porphyria the precursors are found mainly in the urine and faeces. In congenital erythropoietic porphyria the major abnormalities occur in the red blood cells. Biochemical abnormalities are more marked during attacks.

In haem synthesis, two molecules of delta-aminolaevulinic acid (ALA) combine to form a porphobilinogen (PBG) ring. Four rings condense to form uroporphyrinogen, which is converted to coproporphyrinogen, then to protoporphyrin, which combines with iron to form haem.

Urine Delta-Aminolaevulinic Acid (ALA)
Collected in a dark bottle into 10 ml glacial acetic acid and refrigerated.

Normal
10–50 μmol per 24 h

Urine Porphobilinogen (PBG)
Collected into a dark bottle with 5 g sodium carbonate and refrigerated.

Normal
0–10 μmol per 24 h (0–2.0 mg)

Screening test
If PBG is present, a red colour develops when equal parts of fresh urine and Ehrlich's reagent are mixed. If this is shaken with butanol, the red PBG compound enters the upper butanol layer, unlike urobilinogen which stays in the aqueous layer. If excess porphyrins are present, a red fluorescence appears under ultraviolet light when fresh urine or faeces are mixed with an extracting solvent containing equal parts of ether, glacial acetic acid and amyl alcohol.

Uroporphyrin (UP)
Urine is collected into a dark bottle with 5 g sodium carbonate and refrigerated.

Normal 0–60 nmol per 24 h

Normal faecal excretion is 12–48 nmol per 24 h. UP should be absent from heparinized blood.

Coproporphyrin (CP)
Urine is collected into a dark bottle, refrigerated and kept at neutral pH.

Normal 0–0.3 μmol per 24 h

Normal faecal excretion is 600–1800 nmol per 24 h. Heparinized whole blood contains less than 30 nmol/l red cells.

Protoporphyrin (PP)
Faecal excretion is less than 2.7 μmol per 24 h. Specimens should be refrigerated. Heparinized whole blood contains less than 0.9 μmol/l red cells.

Clinical Syndromes

Acute intermittent porphyria
Episodic abdominal pain, with a discrepant absence of abdominal

physical signs but with tachycardia, hypertension, neuropathy or hyponatraemia. Precipitated by drugs. The urine may turn red on standing owing to the conversion of PBG to porphyrin. Urine PBG and ALA are raised.

Porphyria cutanea tarda
Skin rashes exacerbated by sunlight, alcohol and oestrogens. Abnormal liver function tests. No family history. Urine UP and CP and faecal CP and PP are raised.

Acquired porphyrias
These are seen with lead poisoning and liver disease. Photosensitive rashes occur. In lead poisoning, urine ALA and CP rise. In liver disease, urine UP and CP rise, but urine ALA may be normal.

Rare porphyrias
These tend to affect the skin and liver. Red cell studies may be necessary.

WILSON'S DISEASE (WD)

There is a congenital metabolic error affecting the transport and storage of copper. It presents with liver disease, splenomegaly, brain damage or rarely renal disease between the ages of 5 and 50.

Diagnosis is made from the presence of the characteristic corneal Kayser–Fleischer ring, detected by a slit lamp and the serum caeruloplasmin. In difficult cases, serum copper, urine copper and hepatic copper, obtained by liver biopsy, can be measured.

Serum Caeruloplasmin

Normal

Adults	0.9–2.6 μmol/l
Infants	1.0–3.3 μmol/l
Children	2.0–4.3 μmol/l
Pregnancy	higher than normal adult.

The serum level of this copper-binding protein is the best screening test. It is usually low in Wilson's disease, but this may be masked by a rise due to pregnancy, oestrogens or hepatitis.

Other Tests

In Wilson's disease, serum copper is low (normal adult 11–24 μmol/l), urine copper is increased (normal adult 0.24–0.47 μmol per 24 h) and hepatic copper is above 0.55 μmol per gram dry liver. Urinary and hepatic copper may be increased in biliary cirrhosis and rarely cholestasis and other types of cirrhosis, but caeruloplasmin levels are normal or high, not low.

HAEMOCHROMATOSIS

Primary haemochromatosis is a congenital disorder of iron absorption, characterized by the accumulation of iron and its deposition in tissue. It presents mainly with cirrhosis, diabetes, heart disease and skin pigmentation. Secondary haemochromatosis or haemosiderosis is caused by increased iron intake whether oral, parenteral or by blood transfusion. Alcoholic cirrhosis, thalassaemia and sideroblastic anaemia are also associated with iron accumulation. Serum iron is elevated and the TIBC tends to be low and is over 80% saturated. There is increased iron in a liver biopsy. It can be difficult to distinguish primary haemochromatosis from other diseases associated with iron overload, particularly alcoholic cirrhosis. With primary haemochromatosis there may be a family history; excessive iron in a liver biopsy, despite relatively mild cirrhosis and iron deficiency does not appear until at least 10 g of iron has been removed by venesection (40 pints).

Chapter Fourteen

JOINT DISEASE

Diagnosis is essentially clinical, but the tests below may be helpful. Note that a raised ESR suggests inflammatory or systemic disease and that X-ray changes are not seen in the early stages of most diseases.

Rheumatoid Factors (RF)
These are IgM antibodies, appearing in rheumatoid arthritis, which agglutinate red cells or other particles coated with IgG. The distribution of RF titres is a continuous variable in the population and sera are called positive when titres exceed an arbitrary level. Low titre positives are seen in up to 5% of normals and occur more frequently in the elderly, relatives of rheumatoid patients, and in the conditions described below. There are several variations of the test and often the more sensitive they are, the less specific they are.

Serological Tests for Rheumatoid Factor
In the latex fixation test, latex particles are coated with human IgG and agglutinated by serum or joint fluid containing antiglobulin RF. In the Rose–Waaler test (sheep cell agglutination test, SCAT) sheep red cells are sensitized by being coated with rabbit anti-sheep red cell antibody globulin and are similarly agglutinated by RF. Human red cells coated with gamma globulin are also used. The latex test is more sensitive but less specific than the erythrocyte agglutination tests. Tests positive with a greater dilution of serum are more significant. Agglutination at a titre of 1:32 or more is taken as significant in some tests.

Positive tests
1. Rheumatoid arthritis—one or other test is positive in about 70% of patients, especially those with nodules or vasculitis. Early high titres (>1:640) suggest severe disease and a worse prognosis.

Gold or penicillamine may lower titres slowly, but other drugs have less effect. Positive tests in juvenile rheumatoid arthritis suggest a worse prognosis, and they are usually negative in this condition.

2. Sjögren's syndrome—usually positive.
3. Connective tissue disease—SLE, systemic sclerosis, etc. Positive in 10–50%. In SLE, RFs do not usually occur in high titre.
4. Liver disease—cirrhosis, chronic active hepatitis.
5. Diseases with hypergammaglobulinaemia, e.g. sarcoidosis, SBE.

Tests for Systemic Lupus Erythematosus (SLE)
Antibodies occur against many cellular components and also against cells such as red cells, white cells, and platelets. Arthritis without deformity is usual. The demonstration of antibodies against nuclear components or DNA is helpful. The LE cell test is less used now.

Antinuclear Factor/Antibody (ANF/ANA)
This is an immunofluorescent test on serum. Antinuclear gamma globulin autoantibody adsorbs onto the nuclei in a section of unfixed tissue and is identified when fluorescein-labelled antihuman immunoglobulin reacts with it. Positive sera are diluted to determine titre. Chloroquine blocks the ANF reaction. It is the main screening test for SLE, and a negative test almost excludes it. Titres may fall with clinical improvement.

Nuclear fluorescence pattern
The peripheral (rim, shaggy) pattern occurs with antibodies to DNA. The diffuse (homogeneous) pattern reflects antibodies to nucleoprotein. Both are fairly specific for SLE. The speckled pattern reflects antibodies to an extractable nuclear antigen (ENA). The nucleolar pattern is due to antibodies to RNA. Both are less specific for SLE.

High titres ($> 1:50$)
1. SLE.
2. Other connective tissue disorders—Sjögren's syndrome (about 70%); systemic sclerosis (about 50%, often a speckled pattern); rheumatoid arthritis, adult (30%) and juvenile (15%).
3. Other autoimmune disease, e.g. chronic active hepatitis, myasthenia gravis.

4. Drugs (p. 142).

Low titres (< 1:50)
ANF is positive in about 5% of normals, especially the elderly. It also occurs in low titre in the conditions above.

LE Cell Test
IgG antinucleoprotein antibody (LE cell factor) enters a white cell and attacks its nucleus, which loses its chromatin and is extruded as a homogeneous mass (LE body). This body is ingested by a polymorphonuclear cell whose nucleus is pushed to one side by the mass. This is the LE cell. It is less sensitive than the ANF test.

Anti-Deoxyribonucleic Acid (DNA) Antibodies
Antibodies that bind radiolabelled single-stranded, denatured DNA (s-DNA) are present in 90% of patients with SLE, but are also present in several other disorders. Antibodies to native double-stranded DNA (d-DNA) are not so frequently present but are more specific. The radioimmunoassay for d-DNA is the standard serological test for SLE. Levels of over 20 U/ml make the diagnosis likely and the antibody concentration parallels disease activity.

Synovial Fluid
Aspiration under strict asepsis is useful mainly in suspected infection and crystal synovitis. It is particularly indicated in monoarticular effusion. Synovial biopsy may be necessary in tuberculosis. Bacteriological tests should always be done.

Normal fluid—clear, viscous and pale yellow. The mucin clot formed after mixing a few drops of 50% acetic acid with 2–3 ml of fluid is a dense white ball which does not disintegrate on inverting the tube. The cell count is below $1000/mm^3$, mainly mononuclears.
1. Osteoarthritis—the fluid is normal.
2. Active rheumatoid arthritis—the fluid is opalescent or turbid and pale green. The mucin clot is softer and may disintegrate with gentle inversion of the tube. The nucleated cell count is 10 000–50 000/mm^3, often mainly polymorphs. RFs may be found.
3. Septic arthritis—the fluid is opalescent or turbid and there is no mucin clot. The cell count is 10 000–100 000/mm^3, mainly polymorphonuclear, unless the infection is tuberculous. Aspiration should be carried out before antibiotics. If these have been given,

Gram-staining may be positive despite negative culture results. Staining for acid-fast bacilli is mandatory.
4. Crystal synovitis—a clear golden viscous fluid. In gout, birefringent crystals of sodium biurate are seen in the deposit under polarized light. In pseudogout, shorter, broader crystals occur and can be seen in a stained (Romanowsky) smear, which dissolves urate crystals.

Human Leucocyte Antigens (HLA)

These are the main histocompatability antigens and are responsible for graft rejection. They occur in all nucleated cells and are recognized by serological tests in lymphocytes. Their presence is controlled by four gene loci, A, B, C, and D, found on the sixth chromosome. The presence of certain HLA antigens is associated with a tendency to develop certain diseases, possibly because the relevant genes occur close together. Most important clinically is the relationship between HLA-B27 and rheumatic disease.

HLA-B27

It occurs in 8% of normal Europeans, but in 90% of those with ankylosing spondylitis. Its absence makes the diagnosis less likely, but not all who have it develop ankylosing spondylitis. It is also common in other seronegative arthritides and in acute anterior uveitis.

Serum Urate

Normal

Adult male	0.20–0.42 mmol/l
Adult female	
(premenopausal)	0.15–0.36 mmol/l
(postmenopausal)	0.15–0.46 mmol/l
Children	0.12–0.33 mmol/l
Elderly male	0.20–0.47 mmol/l
Pregnancy	reduction by about 30%

Increase

Urate concentration may be raised owing to reduced excretion or increased production. It is measured mainly in the diagnosis of gout.

It is not always raised in this condition and can be high in several other circumstances:

1. Gout (p. 144).
2. Increased production—myeloproliferative disorder, especially myelomatosis and polycythaemia, chronic haemolysis, psoriasis, high-protein diet.
3. Reduced excretion
   (a) Renal failure.
   (b) Hypertension.
   (c) Pre-eclampsia.
   (d) Acidosis, e.g. keto-acidosis and lactic acidosis as in exertion, starvation and disease.
   (e) Hypercalcaemia—hyperparathyroidism, sarcoidosis.
   (f) Myxoedema.
   (g) Drugs—diuretics such as thiazides and frusemide (not spironolactone or amiloride); alcohol; low-dose aspirin. Ethambutol, paracetamol and levodopa may affect measurement.

Effects of increase
Gout is very likely to appear eventually if serum urate levels are maintained over 0.60 mmol/l. Also, uric acid calculi and interstitial nephritis may occur, and treatment is therefore generally indicated. Levels of over 0.90 mmol/l may cause rapid renal damage by tubular blockage.

Decrease
1. Pregnancy—it falls early by about 30%, but tends to rise back towards normal in the last trimester. There is a slight rise in chronic renal disease, but in severe pre-eclampsia it may rise to well above non-pregnant levels.
2. Fanconi syndrome.
3. Drugs—allopurinol, probenecid, aspirin (above 6 g per 24 h), radiocontrast agents, saline infusions, azathioprine, ACTH, coumarin anticoagulants.

CLINICAL PROBLEMS
Connective Tissue Disease
Rheumatoid arthritis, SLE, systemic necrotizing vasculitis, Sjögren's syndrome, systemic sclerosis, dermatomyositis and poly-

myositis are included in this category. Immunological disturbance occurs and the conditions may be related. A raised ESR, polyconal hyperglobulinaemia, anaemia, leucopenia, thrombocytopenia, positive RFs and ANF may be found. The ESR and IgG concentration often parallel disease activity. All except polyarteritis are commoner in women.

Systemic Lupus Erythematosus (SLE)
This disease is commonest in young women. Its manifestations are protean and include vasculitis, arthritis, pleuritis, pericarditis, skin rashes, neuropsychiatric disturbance and nephritis. The liver is not involved.

Diagnostic tests in order of specificity are the anti-DNA antibody test, LE cell test and high titre ANF test, but the sensitivity is in the reverse order. Anti-DNA antibody is high and C4 and C3 levels (p. 19) are particularly likely to be low, with renal involvement and parallel disease activity. Other abnormalities found are a high ESR, anaemia, lymphopenia, mild thrombocytopenia, hyperglobulinaemia, cryoglobulins, immune deposits in the skin, false-positive tests for syphilis, a positive Coomb's test, and an abnormal EEG, with only mild CNS disturbance. RFs may be positive in low titre. CRP levels are raised only if there is infection. SLE is not likely to be present if the ESR is normal and the ANF is negative.

Drug-induced SLE
This is most commonly caused by hydralazine and procainamide and it mimics SLE except that it occurs equally in men, regresses on stopping the drug, does not usually involve the kidneys, and DNA antibodies are not characteristic. It is also seen with reserpine, methyldopa, penicillin, suphonamide, isoniazid, oral contraceptives and phenytoin, among other drugs.

Systemic Necrotizing Vasculitis
The clinical presentation is very varied, although acute illness with arthralgia and myalgia is common. Vasculitic skin rashes, hypertension, mononeuritis multiplex, lung involvement and nephritis frequently occur. Anaemia, leucocytosis and a high ESR are common, and eosinophilia is a suggestive finding. Some abnormality on full urinalysis is often present. Proof can only be by biopsy demonstra-

tion of arteritis or angiographic demonstration of aneurysms. Renal biopsies usually show proliferative glomerulonephritis.

Rheumatoid Arthritis (RA)

This is a subacute or chronic inflammatory polyarthritis involving the peripheral joints, usually with signs of systemic illness. Low titre RFs do not absolutely distinguish rheumatoid disease from osteoarthritis. Persistently negative RFs in a polyarthropathy bring to mind seronegative arthritis. High-titre anti-DNA antibodies are rarely present, but a positive ANF is common. High-titre RFs and severe arthritis favour RA, but a high titre ANF, low-titre RFs and mild arthritis favour SLE.

In active disease there is a high ESR, a high CRP, a low Hb, a low serum iron and a low serum albumin. With improvement, these return towards normal, though sometimes the ESR remains elevated.

The first radiological sign is periarticular osteoporosis, followed by joint-space narrowing and erosions of subchondral bone.

Sjögren's Syndrome

This is a triad of xerostomia (dry mouth), keratoconjunctivitis sicca (dry eyes) and a rheumatic disease. Keratoconjunctivitis and xerostomia alone are called the sicca syndrome. Dryness of the eyes may be demonstrated by Schirmer's test. A strip of filter paper is inserted behind the lower lid of each eye and folded down over the cheek. If less than 5 mm becomes wet, this is abnormal, and if more than 15 mm, it is normal. Most patients show hyperglobulinaemia, antibodies against smooth muscle, gastric parietal cells or thyroid tissue. RFs are usually present, often in high titre even in the absence of rheumatoid disease. ANF may be present.

Systemic Sclerosis

Systemic sclerosis is associated with vascular insufficiency, ischaemic atrophy and fibrosis affecting the skin and viscera, especially the gastrointestinal tract. Raynaud's phenomenon often occurs early. RFs if present are usually in low titre. ANF is more often present and may show a nucleolar or speckled pattern.

Mixed Connective Tissue Disease

There are clinical features of SLE, systemic sclerosis and polymyositis. The serological abnormalities include a positive ANF with a speckled pattern and antibodies to an extractable ribonuclear protein antigen.

Seronegative Arthritis

Ankylosing spondylitis, psoriatic arthropathy, Reiter's syndrome and enteropathic arthropathy come into this group. RFs are absent. The ESR is raised in active disease. The legs, spine and sacro-iliac joints are often affected. HLA-B27 is present in some patients. Ankylosing spondylitis is characterized by inflammation at the sites of attachment of ligaments and joint capsules to bone. Healing is associated with excessive bone formation. It usually presents as low back pain in young males. The spine and costovertebral joints are affected. Iritis and aortitis occur. The first radiological changes are seen in the sacro-iliac joints. The alkaline phosphatase may be raised. In cases of doubt the leucocytes should be examined for HLA-B27, which is present in 90% of patients.

Reiter's syndrome is characterized by a triad of urethritis, arthritis and conjunctivitis in young men. Osteoporosis and periostitis may be seen on X-ray. HLA-B27 is positive in two-thirds of patients.

Psoriatic arthritis differs from RA in being often asymmetrical and involving the distal finger joints and the sacro-iliac joints. Psoriasis of the skin or nails is usually present in the patient or relatives. Enteropathic arthropathy is seen with Crohn's disease and ulcerative colitis. It affects mainly large joints of the legs.

Polymyalgia Rheumatica

Pain and stiffness of the proximal extremities and torso, worse in the morning, affects patients over 50 years old. The ESR is almost always over 40 mm/l per h. Values between 30 and 40 mm/l per h should be checked. RFs are negative. The response to prednisolone 20 mg daily is rapid.

Gout

Gout is caused by the deposition of uric acid crystals in joints and other tissues. It is an acute recurrent monoarthritis, with severe pain, redness and swelling developing within a few hours and subsiding within a week. It often affects the first metatarsophalangeal joint in males and postmenopausal females. Chronic gout with tophi, renal calculi and nephritis may follow. Cellulitis, septic arthritis, pseudogout, traumatic synovitis and bunions should be considered in the differential diagnosis.

The serum urate will always be raised on repeated measurement unless treatment has been given (p. 140). Synovial fluid examination reveals uric acid crystals in cases of doubt. Pseudogout involves large joints, causes articular calcification and is associated with pyrophosphate crystals in the synovial fluid.

Chapter Fifteen

DISEASES OF THE GUT AND PANCREAS

OESOPHAGUS

Preliminary investigation is by the radiological screening of swallowed barium. This reveals major pathology, e.g. carcinoma, hiatus hernia, achalasia, strictures and pouches. Endoscopy, with biopsy when indicated, gives evidence of oesophagitis and varices.

Other techniques used in the investigation of obscure chest pain and oesophageal motility disorders include isotope methods to study reflux, manometry for spasm and acid perfusion studies. Through a nasal tube 0.1 mol/l hydrochloric acid, 0.1 mol/l sodium bicarbonate and then normal saline are run into the oesophagus at a rate of 10 ml/min., changing the solution without informing the patient. The test is positive if acid provokes the usual pain in ten minutes and bicarbonate relieves it.

STOMACH AND DUODENAL CAP

The anatomy is demonstrated by barium studies. Endoscopy enables inspection of the mucosa and samples can be taken for histology.

Barium Meal
This is positive in 90% of patients with duodenal ulcer in most centres. A deformed duodenal cap confirms previous, and is consistent with current, ulceration, but scarring makes active ulcers hard to see. Superficial lesions are not well shown even with double contrast studies. Appearances are more difficult to interpret after

surgery. The suspected clinical diagnosis must be indicated, as this affects the radiological technique.

Endoscopy

This supplements the barium meal, but in acute bleeding it is the investigation of choice, as the source of bleeding can be located. It may reveal superficial lesions, e.g. mucosal tears, inflammation, acute erosions and varices. Active ulceration in a deformed duodenal cap or stomal ulcers may be shown. Histology can be obtained and this is especially important when malignancy is considered.

Gastric Aspiration Tests

Acid output is proportional to pepsin output, but these tests are usually unhelpful in peptic ulcer problems because of the overlap with normal. They are used in suspected gastrinoma and to distinguish appropriate from inappropriate fasting hypergastrinaemia. They can also be used to test the adequacy of a vagotomy. Fasting volume, basal secretion and peak acid output are determined. Fifteen minute aliquots are taken.

Normal

1. Fasting volume (early morning aspirate)—this is normally below 50 ml. Volumes of over 200 ml indicate marked gastric retention and volumes of between 50 and 200 ml are consistent with mild retention or hypersecretion. The test is useful in the assessment of pyloric stenosis.
2. Basal acid output (BAO)—normal 0–5 mmol/h.
3. Maximal stimulation (peak acid output, PAO)—the output in the peak 30 minutes after pentagastrin 6 μg/kg is multiplied by two.
   Normal: Males   1–40 mmol/h.
               Females   1–30 mmol/h.

Serum Gastrin

Normal

Adults: < 100 ng/l (may be higher in elderly).
Serum gastrin levels are measured on three fasting samples in aggressive peptic ulcer disease, and if the Zollinger–Ellison syn-

drome (ZES) is present, at least one will show marked, inappropriate elevation, i.e. despite hyperchlorhydria. Inappropriate elevation also occurs in gastric retention and antral G-cell hyperplasia. Appropriate elevation, due to low or absent acid secretion, occurs in gastric atrophy, pernicious anaemia and post vagotomy, and high levels occur in renal failure.

ZES is characterized by severe peptic ulcer disease, with recurrent ulceration, sometimes in atypical sites, and sometimes with diarrhoea. It is caused by a non-beta cell tumour of the pancreatic islets (gastrinoma). Gastric aspiration studies show a basal volume of over 200 ml/h, a BAO of over 15 mmol/h and more than 40% of the PAO (normal below 20%). After gastric surgery, aspiration tests are not reliable and in any case ZES must be confirmed by gastrin levels.

X-Ray Negative Dyspepsia
If adequate radiology and endoscopy are negative, peptic ulcer disease is unlikely, but if there is doubt, a therapeutic trial may be undertaken. If symptoms do not subside with bed rest in hospital and active medical treatment, uncomplicated peptic ulcer disease is unlikely. Other pathologies may temporarily respond. Biliary tract disease, pancreatitis, Meckel's diverticulum, irritable bowel syndrome, mesenteric ischaemia and porphyria should be considered.

MALABSORPTION AND THE SMALL BOWEL

Malabsorption is often but not exclusively due to disease of the small bowel. Small bowel disease commonly causes malabsorption, but can present with pain or other symptoms. Malabsorption can cause steatorrhoea, nutritional defects or both. Steatorrhoea is often, but not always, associated with increased frequency of bowel movement. The anatomy of the small bowel is studied by barium and its histology by jejunal biopsy. The best initial tests to establish the presence of malabsorption are faecal fat excretion and xylose absorption. Low serum carotene levels are common.

Common causes of malabsorption
1. Structural lesions—gastric surgery, intestinal resection, Crohn's disease, blind loops, diverticula, fistulae, partial obstruction.

2. Mucosal abnormalities—gluten enteropathy, tropical sprue, Whipple's disease, alactasia.
3. Pancreatic disease (see below).
4. Biliary disease.
5. Infection—acute enteritis, tuberculosis, parasites, e.g. giardiasis.
6. Iatrogenic—phenindione, neomycin, abdominal radiotherapy.
7. Primarily non gastrointestinal disease—malignancy, severe skin disease (dermatitis herpetiformis), hyperthyroidism, systemic sclerosis.

In the United Kingdom gluten enteropathy is the commonest cause, followed by Crohn's disease, then chronic pancreatitis. Malabsorption due to gastric surgery is common but mild.

Barium Studies
A barium follow-through may show flocculation and absence of mucosal pattern in any form of steatorrhoea. Non-flocculating barium shows the anatomy better. A small bowel enema involves direct filling of the duodenum with a small volume of dilute barium and gives a better picture. A barium enema may show ileocaecal pathology best.

Jejunal Biopsy
This is very helpful in the diagnosis of mucosal abnormalities, but as only one site is usually sampled it can miss patchy lesions and does not reveal the extent of disease. Also, in many conditions the response of the mucosa is a non-specific villous atrophy.
1. Gluten enteropathy—subtotal villous atrophy. Response to gluten withdrawal.
2. Tropical sprue (TS)—a variable villous atrophy, less severe than in gluten enteropathy, occurs. TS is defined as malabsorption of at least two unrelated substances in someone who has visited the tropics. There is usually steatorrhoea and folate deficiency, with a response to tetracycline.
3. Specific abnormalities—these are all rare and include amyloidosis, lymphoma, lymphangiectasia and Whipple's disease.
4. Dermatogenic enteropathy—in dermatitis herpetiformis, partial

villous atrophy responsive to gluten withdrawal occurs, and atrophy also occurs in other extensive skin diseases.
5. Giardiasis (p. 88).

Faecal Fat

Normal
Adults $<$ 18 mmol per 24 h.
Children (up to 6 years) $<$ 7 mmol per 24 h.

The standard collection is for three, preferably five, days on a normal diet containing at least 50 g of fat daily. Excretion of between 18 and 25 mmol per 24 h is equivocal. Mild cases may be detected by seven days collection on a diet containing 100 g of fat, over 7% of which is excreted.

Fat is absorbed mainly in the midgut. Visible oil or fat in the stool is usually due to pancreatic disease.

Xylose Tolerance Test

The fasting patient takes xylose 5 g (33 mmol) and urine is collected for 5 hours. Whole blood specimens are taken in a fluoride tube.

Normal

Adults	Urine excretion of over 8 mmol per 5 h and blood level (at 2 hours) of over 1.7 mmol/l.
Children	Urine excretion of over 16% of ingested dose and blood level (at 1 hour) of over 2.0 mmol/l.

Unless there is renal failure, urine output is more reliable than blood levels, as the latter fluctuate. Blood levels below 0.7 mmol/l indicate malabsorption and values between 0.7 and 1.7 mmol/l are equivocal. Xylose is absorbed from the duodenum and upper jejunum and absorption is usually normal in disease of the stomach, pancreas, liver and ileum. Abnormality occurs especially in gluten enteropathy, but also when the jejunum is involved in diverticulosis, Crohn's disease and Whipple's disease. False-positives occur as below:

1. Reduced absorption—pernicious anaemia, Parkinsonism, indomethacin treatment.

2. Sequestration of xylose—oedema and ascites.
3. Reduced excretion (blood levels are usually normal, but urine output is low). In elderly patients, renal failure, aspirin treatment, or poor bladder emptying.

Lactose Tolerance Test
The test is performed with 75 g lactose as for a standard glucose tolerance test (OGTT).

Abnormal result
1. The blood glucose rises by less than 1.2 mmol/l after lactose.
2. There is a normal rise in blood glucose and no symptoms, with an OGTT done on a different day.
3. The patient's symptoms, usually watery stools, flatus and abdominal distension, are reproduced.

Causes of lactose intolerance
1. Isolated lactose deficiency. This may present in infancy or adult life, with symptoms as indicated above. The intestinal mucosa is normal. There may be a mild associated steatorrhoea. The condition may be asymptomatic or it may clinically resemble the irritable bowel syndrome. It is commoner in non-Caucasians.
2. Secondary to mucosal disease, e.g. gluten enteropathy or gastroenteritis.

The radioactive-carbon breath test is usually also abnormal and low lactose activity is found in a jejunal biopsy specimen. The stool may have a pH of as low as 4.0 in a disaccharidase deficiency, whereas it is normally 7.0.

Tests for Bacterial Overgrowth
This is often associated with a radiologically demonstrable bowel lesion or stasis.

Indican in urine
Abnormal bacteria in the jejunum break down tryptophan to indole, which is excreted as indican.

Normal
10–80 mg per 24 h

A slight increase ($<$ 100 mg per 24 h) is seen in any disease of the small bowel mucosa. A marked increase ($>$ 150 mg per 24 h) suggests the presence of abnormal small bowel bacteria. The test is not very reliable. Excretion is decreased in pancreatic disease.

Jejunal aspiration
Jejunal fluid aspiration should normally reveal only oropharyngeal organisms in a concentration of below 10^5/ml. In bacterial overgrowth, bacteroides and other aerobic and anaerobic gut organisms may be discovered in a concentration of over 10^6/ml.

Carbon-14 bile salt breath test
Bile salts from the liver facilitate fat absorption in the jejunum, are reabsorbed in the ileum and are recirculated. Fat malabsorption therefore occurs with hepatic cirrhosis, cholestasis, ileal disease, and also with bacterial contamination of the jejunum. In the last case, bacteria deconjugate and therefore inactivate the bile salts. A conjugated bile salt is given with the amino acid labelled by carbon-14. In the presence of bacteria in the jejunum, deconjugation occurs, the amino-acid is absorbed and radioactive carbon dioxide can be detected in the breath. With ileal disease, the unabsorbed bile salt is deconjugated by colonic bacteria and is similarly detected.

Therapeutic response
There is clinical improvement with broad-spectrum antibiotics.

Schilling Test (p. 250)
Abnormality is corrected by intrinsic factor in gastric disease and by broad-spectrum antibiotics in bacterial overgrowth, but cannot be corrected in ileal disease.

Oral Glucose Tolerance Test (OGTT)
Glucose is absorbed mainly in the jejunum and the OGTT may be diabetic in pancreatic disease, oxyhyperglycaemic (lag storage) after gastrectomy, and flat in other types of malabsorption.

Tests for Protein Loss

Faecal nitrogen content may increase owing to malabsorption or protein-losing enteropathy. It is normally below 40 mmol per 24 h in infants and below 140 mmol per 24 h in adults.

Protein loss from the gut can be demonstrated by measuring the appearance of injected radiochromium-labelled albumin in the stool. It occurs in various mucosal and other gut diseases. It may present as hypoalbuminaemia, without obvious cause.

Tests for Nutritional Deficiencies

The detection of nutritional deficiencies provides confirmation that there is malabsorption, gives some evidence about its cause, and is

important for treatment. Deficiencies of calories, protein, haematinics, vitamins and minerals occur (see Chapter 6). Deficiencies may be aggravated by poor intake. Serum albumin and cholesterol levels can be reduced in malabsorption of most types.

Anaemia

The haemoglobin is usually normal in pancreatic disease. The serum iron is most likely to fall in gastric and duodenal disease. Folate deficiency is associated especially with jejunal disease. The serum B12 may be low in gastric and ileal disease, and bacterial overgrowth.

Vitamins

Serum carotene levels are low, especially in small bowel disease. The prothrombin time may be prolonged due to vitamin K deficiency. Vitamin D deficiency causes osteomalacia.

Minerals

Serum calcium and magnesium levels may be low.

MISCELLANEOUS

Stool Examination

Microscopy of saline emulsion

Pus and blood are found in ulcerative colitis and some infective diarrhoeas. Fat droplets and fatty acid crystals may be seen in steatorrhoea. Mature parasites and ova are sought when infestations such as hookworm, amoebiasis and giardiasis are suspected.

Stool culture
This is essential in acute and chronic diarrhoea. The isolation of tubercle bacilli is difficult but particularly relevant in Asian patients.

Occult blood
Most tests exploit the pseudoperoxidase activity of haemoglobin. Serial tests must be done to improve the chance of picking up a lesion which bleeds intermittently. Bleeding from oral, nasal and anal sources and drug-induced bleeding must be excluded. Strongly positive and repeatedly negative tests give useful information. Weak positive tests require careful evaluation. The exclusion of dietary meat and toothbrushing may help to settle their significance.

Ascitic Fluid

Cells
A blood-stained fluid suggests malignancy or tuberculosis. Cytology may reveal malignant cells.

Chemistry
A transudate with a protein content of below 20 g/l is associated with generalized fluid retention. An exudate with a protein content of above 30 g/l is found in peritonitis, malignancy and hepatic vein thrombosis. The protein content can be high in cirrhosis. A high lactate dehydrogenase level suggests malignancy. The amylase concentration is raised in pancreatitis and perforated peptic ulcer.

Culture
This is mandatory with any paracentesis and unexpected tuberculous or other infection may be discovered.

Urine 5-Hydroxyindole-Acetic Acid (5-HIAA)

Normal
10–45 μmol per 24 h.

Screening test—random urine specimen turns purple with nitroso-naphthal. Carcinoid tumour tissue metabolizes dietary tryptophan to serotonin, which causes alimentary hyperperistalsis and bronchial constriction. Serotonin is further metabolized to 5-HIAA. Very high excretion rates occur in carcinoid syndrome and slightly raised excretion may occur with other neoplasms and steatorrhoea. Seroto-nin-rich foods such as bananas cause false-positives. Phenothiazines cause false negatives.

PANCREAS

Imaging
The gland is deep in the abdomen and is difficult to study—especially the body and tail. Plain X-ray reveals calcification, ultrasound may show cysts or masses and barium meals including hypotonic duodenography may demonstrate the pancreatic head.

Computerized tomography is usually the next examination consi-dered. Isotope scans are often difficult to interpret. The invasive investigations which may be necessary are angiography for tumours and endoscopic retrograde cholangiopancreatography (ERCP) for pancreatitis.

Serum Amylase

Normal

Adults	70–200 IU/l
Elderly	slightly higher values may be normal.

Amylase levels are usually measured in the investigation of acute abdominal pain.

Increase
1. Acute pancreatitis—the level may start to rise within three hours of the onset, peaks at 24 hours and often returns to normal within 72 hours. Blood should therefore be taken on admission and the next day. Only levels over three times normal are strongly suggestive. The rise may be reduced or absent if blood is taken shortly after food, during glucose infusion, with overwhelming attacks or in recurrent acute pancreatitis. Elevation for more than

seven days suggests a severe attack and persistence for more than 14 days suggests pseudocyst formation or pancreatic ascites.

2. Other abdominal emergencies—perforated peptic ulcer, obstruction of the efferent loop of a Polya gastrectomy, and mesenteric infarction may cause high levels owing to absorption of amylase from the gut. Several other acute abdominal conditions, e.g. cholecystitis and ruptured aneurysm, can cause a modest and sometimes a marked rise in amylase, because of secondary pancreatic involvement.

3. Drug-induced—any drug which can cause pancreatic duct obstruction, pancreatitis or parotitis, e.g. opiates, thiazides, corticosteroids, phenylbutazone and after cholecystography.

4. Persistent increase without abdominal symptoms
   (a) Renal failure by itself can raise the level to twice normal and exacerbates a rise from other causes.
   (b) Salivary gland disease—persistent asymptomatic hyperamylasaemia is usually of salivary origin, even if the salivary glands are normal.
   (c) Metastatic tumours.
   (d) Macroamylasaemia.

Urine Amylase

Normal
127–1310 IU/l (lower in neonates)

Ratio clearance of amylase: clearance of creatinine 1–4%

$$\frac{\text{Urine amylase}}{\text{Serum amylase}} \times \frac{\text{Serum creatinine}}{\text{Urine creatinine}} \times 100$$

Urinary amylase is a more sensitive and persistent (up to 10 days) indicator of acute pancreatitis, but may be normal when there is renal failure. In unexplained hyperamylasaemia a normal clearance ratio suggests a salivary origin and a very low ratio occurs with macroamylasaemia.

Pancreatic Function Tests

Lundh test
A tube is passed in the fasting patient and sited distal to duodeno-jejunal flexure by fluoroscopy. A 400 ml meal of corn oil, skimmed milk powder and dextrose is given and pancreatic juice is collected for two hours. Tryptic activity in the fluid is normally over 25 IU/ml.

Secretin-pancreozymin test
This requires a double lumen tube, with one orifice in the stomach and one in the duodenum. Bicarbonate excretion falls in chronic pancreatitis and enzyme concentration falls, particularly in cancer.

Para-aminobenzoic acid test (PABA)
Radio-labelled PABA is taken with an unlabelled PABA precursor, normally split to release PABA by pancreatic chymotrypsin. In pancreatic disease the urinary excretion of unlabelled PABA is reduced relative to labelled PABA.

PANCREATIC DISEASES

Acute Pancreatitis
Confirmatory tests include serum and urine amylase tests. One may also find hypocalcaemia after the third day, in association with hypoalbuminaemia, hyperglycaemia, jaundice and methaem-albuminaemia. The main causes are biliary disease and alcoholism, rarely hypercalcaemia and hyperlipidaemia and drugs. It is often idiopathic.

Chronic Pancreatitis
In severe disease there is steatorrhoea, impaired glucose tolerance and sometimes pancreatic calcification on plain X-ray. In malabsorption there is usually no anaemia and xylose tolerance is normal. Known causes are alcoholism, biliary disease, hyperlipidaemia, hypercalcaemia and haemochromatosis. Pancreatic function tests and imaging techniques may be necessary, as outlined above. Amylase studies are only useful in acute exacerbations of chronic disease.

Carcinoma

When situated in the head it presents with jaundice, when more distal with pain and weight loss. Ultrasound followed by CT or ERCP are necessary. Percutaneous aspiration of the pancreas for cytology is possible.

Chapter Sixteen

DISEASES OF THE LIVER AND BILIARY TRACT

IMAGING

Plain Abdominal X-Ray
About 10% of gallstones are visible. Liver calcification may be seen.

Oral Cholecystography (OC)
This technique demonstrates stones in a functioning gallbladder and failure to visualize the gallbladder is presumptive evidence of cystic duct obstruction. There are several other reasons why the gallbladder may not be shown, including not taking or vomiting the tablets, malabsorption, parenchymal liver disease, and a raised bilirubin level. A bilirubin concentration of over 30 μmol/l is a contraindication to the technique. Because of the high percentage of misleading results, absence of function should be checked by ultrasound or intravenous cholangiography (IVC). Also, if the OC is normal but stones are still suspected clinically, they may be shown by ultrasound or IVC.

Intravenous Cholangiography
This can demonstrate the bile ducts as well as the gallbladder. It is most useful after cholecystectomy and when the cholecystogram has shown no opacification. It will, however, also be unsuccessful at bilirubin levels of over 50 μmol/l and in the presence of severe liver disease. Dilated ducts suggest present or recent obstruction to the system, even if the pathology is not positively demonstrated. In acute abdominal pain a normal gallbladder shadow is good evidence against cholecystitis, whereas an absent gallbladder shadow, despite good duct visualization, favours it. With inpatients it may be preferable to carry out cholangiography rather than initial cholecystography.

159

Computerized Tomography (CT)

CT is an excellent but expensive technique for detecting space-occupying lesions and determining their nature. In diffuse liver disease an increased fat or iron content may be demonstrated. In jaundice the nature of the obstruction is more likely to be demonstrated than by ultrasound.

Ultrasound

This is a useful means of safely imaging the liver and biliary tract. Space-occupying lesions are well shown and cysts can be distinguished from solid tumours. In cirrhosis, ultrasound is useful to detect ascites, splenomegaly and portal vein dilatation.

Gallstones and thickening of the gallbladder wall can be detected when these cannot be demonstrated by contrast studies.

Jaundice

Ultrasound is the preferred initial imaging technique in the investigation of jaundice. Real-time scanning, in particular, is a sensitive and specific technique for the detection of dilatation of the intra- and extrahepatic biliary tract. It may be possible to locate the site of an obstruction. False-positives and false-negatives can occur if dilatation is mild, however, and in these circumstances the test should be repeated after an interval.

Isotope Scan

Space-occupying lesions

Technetium-labelled colloid, which is taken up by the reticulo-endothelial system will demonstrate most lesions more than 2 cm in diameter. False-negatives occur with deep intrahepatic lesions and false-positives occur in cirrhosis and at the hilum in obstructive jaundice. Abscesses, cysts and tumours are not distinguished, but a gallium scan will fill in an abscess or tumour.

Jaundice

Iminodiacetic acid is taken up by the hepatocytes and excreted like bilirubin. The liver is shown in 10 minutes and the biliary tract and gallbladder in an hour. Delay occurs with obstructive and hepatocellular disease. With complete obstruction activity never reaches the gut. It has poor distinguishing power in jaundice in general, but in acute abdominal conditions failure to demonstrate the gallbladder in an hour is good evidence of cholecystitis.

Cirrhosis
The typical technetium scan shows patchy uptake by the liver and increased uptake by the spleen.

LIVER BIOPSY

This is of especial value in the assessment of chronic hepatitis. It is also useful in the study of cirrhosis, alcoholism, hepatomegaly and splenomegaly. Discrete malignant lesions may be missed, but diffuse disease will be demonstrated by an adequate sample. In systemic conditions such as tuberculosis and sarcoidosis, granulomas may be found and liver biopsy is sometimes useful in pyrexia of unknown origin. The biopsy often shows non-specific changes when it is performed to elucidate relatively minor changes in liver function tests.

LIVER FUNCTION TESTS

Serum Bilirubin

Normal

Adults	3–17 μmol/l
Neonates	< 200 μmol/l in first week
Conjugated bilirubin	2–5 μmol/l

Bilirubin formed by haemoglobin breakdown is conjugated by liver cells to form a water-soluble compound and excreted in the bile. Conjugated or direct-reacting bilirubin is measured by the formation of a diazo dye and total bilirubin from the further colour developed after alcohol is added. Unconjugated or indirect-reacting bilirubin represents the difference between the two readings. Clinically obvious jaundice (bilirubin > 35 μmol/l) is due to liver or biliary disease or haemolysis. Haemolysis is associated with unconjugated hyperbilirubinaemia and biliary obstruction with an increase in the conjugated level. However, bilirubin fractions do not clearly disting-uish biliary obstruction from hepatocellular disease, as obstruction causes liver damage and liver damage causes small duct obstruction, so that in both conditions there is an increase in both fractions.

Unconjugated Bilirubin

In a pure unconjugated hyperbilirubinaemia, the total bilirubin level is below 85 μmol/l, less than 20% of the total is conjugated and there is no bilirubin in the urine. Urine urobilinogen may be increased also.

Increase
1. Haemolysis.
2. Cardiovascular—cardiac failure causes hepatic congestion. It is also often associated with pulmonary infarction, which increases the bilirubin load on the liver.
3. Tissue damage—infarctions and haematoma absorption, especially in children.
4. Non-specific illness—a slight risk often occurs with inflammation, infection and neoplasm.
5. Persistent hyperbilirubinacmia—some represent the tail end of the normal distribution and some Gilbert's or rarer congenital syndromes. If the concentration is below 50 μmol/l and examination, liver function tests and tests for haemolysis are persistently negative, further investigation can be avoided. In Gilbert's syndrome the bilirubin level rises with fasting.

Urine Bilirubin

This is measured by the formation of a diazo dye when a dipstick or tablet, Ictotest (Ames) is impregnated with fresh urine. The tablet test is more sensitive and specific; the dipstick may give a false-positive with chlorpromazine. As bilirubin only appears in the urine when there is obstruction to the excretion of conjugated bilirubin, a positive test indicates hepatobiliary disease. It is a sensitive test which may be positive before the serum bilirubin rises. If it is positive in an obscure illness, hepatic involvement may be suspected. Conversely, a negative test in moderate jaundice suggests unconjugated hyperbilirubinaemia.

Urine Urobilinogen

Normal
50–500 μmol per 24 h; 0.5–4.0 Ehrlich units per 24 h.

Ehrlich's reagent is used. A red colour forms which can be distinguished from porphobilinogen (p. 134).

Screening test
Normal: 0.1–1.0 Ehrlich units per 100 ml.

Urine is tested by a dipstick, Urobilistix (Ames). The urine must be fresh, as on standing urobilinogen breaks down to urobilin, which has the same significance but is measured differently (with zinc acetate). Bilirubin is broken down by gut bacteria to urobilinogen, reabsorbed and recirculated by the liver, with some spilling over into the urine.

Increase
1. Bilirubin production increased—haemolysis, haematoma, absorption and infarction. The unconjugated bilirubin level may rise.
2. Hepatocellular disease—reabsorbed urobilinogen cannot be re-circulated and a positive test may precede hyperbilirubinaemia in hepatitis.
3. Non-specific—fever, constipation, strongly alkaline urine.
4. False-positives—sulphonamides, PAS, phenothiazines.

Decrease
Detection of this requires quantitative measurement.
1. Complete biliary obstruction—persistent absence suggests neo-plastic obstruction and conversely the presence of urobilinogen excludes total biliary obstruction.
2. Gut disturbance—diarrhoea, antibiotics.
3. Renal—acid or stale urine, renal failure.

Serum Alkaline Phosphatase (SAP)
SAP (p. 22) is more sensitive than bilirubin to minor degrees of intra- or extrahepatic obstruction, but is less affected by pure liver cell damage. A rise in the SAP without jaundice is also characteristic of obstruction to a branch of the common bile duct and a very high SAP but a normal serum bilirubin is often seen with metastatic liver disease.

Alkaline phosphatase of bony origin must be distinguished (see below).

Hepatic causes of increase
1. Cholestasis—the higher the SAP level, the more likely is jaundice to be obstructive than hepatic, and vice versa. A level more than

twice normal is an approximate dividing line, but this does not distinguish between intra- and extrahepatic obstruction.
2. Hepatitis—the level is usually less than two-and-a-half times the upper limit of normal.
3. Cholangitis.
4. Space-occupying lesions—carcinoma, abscess, cyst.
5. Hepatic infiltrations—tuberculosis, sarcoidosis.

Alternative enzymes

5'-Nucleotidase (5'-NT) comes only from the liver and is especially useful in the evaluation of liver disease in pregnancy and childhood. A normal level does not completely exclude a hepatic origin for a raised SAP, as the test is slightly less sensitive. Gamma-glutamyltransferase is an alternative to 5'-NT. If these enzymes are normal, a raised SAP probably is of bony origin. The heat stability of SAP will also decide this point.

Serum Gamma-Glutamyltransferase (γ-GT)

This is a sensitive but non-specific test for liver disease (p. 24). It rises to very high levels in cholestasis and also very early in viral and toxic hepatitis, primary biliary cirrhosis, metastatic liver disease, and alcoholism.

Serum Aminotransferases (p. 23)

Aspartate aminotransferase is slighly more sensitive in some kinds of liver disease than alanine aminotransferase, but it is also less specific, as more of it comes from the heart. Both tests are rather non-specific, as levels rise with extensive damage to any tissue. They are useful in liver disease as follows (see p. 23 for normal values):
1. Acute diffuse hepatocellular damage—levels of over 1000 IU/l suggest this and are found in viral hepatitis, toxic damage and ischaemia.
2. Chronic hepatitis—levels persistently over 150 IU/l are suggestive of this whether it be chronic active, chronic persistent, protracted acute viral or drug-induced hepatitis.
3. Viral hepatitis—raised levels confirm anicteric and preicteric cases and can indicate relapse during convalescence. The levels are maximal just after the onset of jaundice.
4. Cholestasis—levels over 400 IU/l, and especially over 1000 IU/l, favour acute parenchymal disease and levels below 100 IU/l

favour obstructive disease. After obstruction has been present for a few weeks enzyme levels rise towards 400 IU/l, and conversely, in the later cholangiolitic stage of hepatitis, enzyme levels fall and a picture of obstruction is left. Blood should therefore be taken early.

5. Early disease—a rise in levels may be an early sign of damage by drugs or infiltration by carcinoma.

Prothrombin Time
This may be prolonged due either to hepatocellular failure or biliary obstruction. An improvement in the prothrombin time 24 hours after vitamin K 10 mg i.v. suggests that jaundice is obstructive and not due to parenchymal disease.

Serum Proteins
These are neither sensitive nor specific indicators of liver disease, but certain patterns are recognized. In acute disease, albumin and α-globulin fall. An albumin concentration of below 30 g/l and a rise in β- and γ-globulin suggest chronic disease. With cholestasis, β- and γ_2-globulins rise. In cirrhosis, albumin falls and γ-globulin rises, sometimes with a fusion of the β and γ globulin peaks. In biliary cirrhosis, β-globulin and α_2-globulin are likely to rise.

Antimitochondrial Antibody (AMA)
This is a fluorescent antibody test, almost always positive in biliary cirrhosis. It is occasionally positive in chronic active hepatitis, cryptogenic cirrhosis and viral hepatitis. In jaundice, a positive test suggests primary biliary cirrhosis, especially when it is of slow onset in a middle-aged woman.

Smooth Muscle Antibody (SMA)
This antibody which reacts against the membrane of most cells is found in many patients with chronic active hepatitis and cirrhosis. It is also positive, however, in infectious mononucleosis and various malignancies.

Immunology in Diagnosis
In acute infective hepatitis, IgM levels rise and IgA and IgG levels may do so also. C3 and C4 levels (p. 18) may be low in the early stages. SMA may appear transiently. HBsAg (p. 83) is usually

positive in hepatitis B. In chronic persistent hepatitis, Ig levels and C3 levels are normal, auto-antibodies are absent. In chronic active hepatitis (CAH), IgG levels are elevated, C3 and C4 levels may be low, and SMA, ANF and AMA may occur. HBsAg may be positive. Younger patients with CAH tend to be female, HBsAg negative and have markedly abnormal IgG levels and auto-antibodies.

Patients with primary biliary cirrhosis (PBC) have high IgM levels, normal IgG and IgA levels and strongly positive AMA. In alcoholic and cryptogenic cirrhosis, IgA, in particular, tends to be elevated. SMA and AMA may be weakly positive in cryptogenic cirrhosis.

CLINICAL PROBLEMS

The Differential Diagnosis of Jaundice

Unconjugated hyperbilirubinaemia can be readily excluded (p. 162), but it may be difficult to decide whether jaundice is hepatocellular or cholestatic. In hepatocellular jaundice, urobilinogen is present in the urine, aminotransferases and plasma proteins may be very abnormal and SAP is not very high. The major causes are hepatitis (p. 82), drugs, cirrhosis and alcoholism.

Deep jaundice may be clearly obstructive, as shown by pruritus, pale stools, dark urine and a high SAP, but the distinction must then be made between intrahepatic (medical) and extrahepatic (surgical) cholestasis, as follows:

1. The clinical evidence must be carefully reassessed and the drug history is particularly important. Simpler imaging studies suffice where extrahepatic obstruction is unlikely and may do so where it is certain. More invasive studies are performed where there is clinical doubt.

2. Imaging techniques—ultrasound is the most useful preliminary test. It will usually distinguish medical from surgical jaundice, but often does not show the cause of the obstruction. A plain abdominal radiograph may show gallstones but they are not necessarily the cause of the obstruction. Isotope studies are often unhelpful, as are barium studies, though a gastric carcinoma or pancreatic lesion may be shown. Computerized tomography is a useful supplement to ultrasound. If it is necessary, the biliary tract can be directly visualized by fine-needle percutaneous cholangiography or endoscopic retrograde cholangiopancreatography.

3. Laboratory tests—they provide cumulative evidence rather than single absolute answers. They should be taken as soon as possible because with time, evidence of a primary hepatitis disappears and evidence of liver damage appears in extrahepatic obstruction. Enzyme levels, SAP, proteins, prothrombin time, AMA, HBsAg (p. 83) and urinary urobilinogen are discussed elsewhere. Note the significance of a persistently absent urinary urobilinogen (p. 162). A positive HBsAg test certainly favours hepatitis, but a patient might be a symptomless carrier with surgical obstruction.
4. Liver biopsy—this may be carried out if the bile ducts are not dilated, but it is often unhelpful.

Causes of Cholestasis

Medical (1–5 intrahepatic)
1. Viral hepatitis (cholangiolitic stage).
2. Drug induced (see below).
3. Cirrhosis—mainly primary biliary, but also cryptogenic cirrhosis.
4. Alcoholic hepatitis.
5. Chronic active hepatitis.
6. Sclerosing cholangitis—presents with progressive obstructive jaundice due to inflammatory thickening of the bile duct. Diagnosis is by the exclusion of other causes, cholangiography and laparotomy.

Surgical (extrahepatic)
1. Gallstones.
2. Neoplasms—affecting the pancreas, the biliary tree or lymph nodes.
3. Stricture.
4. Chronic pancreatitis.

Cirrhosis
This is diagnosed by a combination of the clinical findings, laboratory tests and liver histology.

It is usual to do tests for hepatitis A & B (p. 83); immunoglobulin levels (p. 166); serum ferritin and serum iron and iron-binding capacity (haemochromatosis, p. 136); serum caeruloplasmin (Wilson's disease, p. 135); autoantibodies (primary biliary cirrhosis and chronic active hepatitis); α-fetoprotein (primary hepatoma); serum α_1-antitrypsin (p. 20).

Portal hypertension is suggested by splenomegaly and varices are confirmed by barium swallow or oesophagoscopy. Serum albumin and bilirubin levels indicate the severity of damage in the absence of cholestasis. Aminotransferase levels over 150 IU/l and globulin levels exceeding albumin suggest active disease. Coma is likely to be of hepatic origin if the EEG shows a specific abnormality, characterized by a slow dominant rhythm, and the blood ammonia concentration may be over 80 µmol/l (normal < 20 µmol/l). The prothrombin time is considerably prolonged. The liver biopsy may be helpful in the diagnosis of biliary cirrhosis, chronic active hepatitis, alcoholic disease, haemochromatosis and Wilson's disease.

Drugs and the Liver
The liver metabolizes drugs to water-soluble compounds which are excreted by the kidney. Adverse drug reactions are common.

Enzyme induction
The microsomal enzymes are stimulated by drugs such as barbiturates, phenytoin, alcohol, rifampicin and dichloralphenazone. This increases the metabolism of other drugs, reducing their effects. The γ-GT level rises, but there is no liver damage.

Pure cholestasis
A marked rise in serum bilirubin may be seen with synthetic oestrogens and androgens, rifampicin and sodium fusidate. Other liver function tests are relatively normal.

Dose-dependent toxicity
Hepatic necrosis is seen with paracetamol and iron poisoning, high-dose tetracycline and, in mild form, with high-dose salicylates. Azathioprine and methotrexate also cause hepatic toxicity.

Idiosyncratic reactions
Histologically and clinically, hepatitis, hepatic necrosis or cholestasis may predominate. The drug has usually been started within the last few months and there is improvement on withdrawal, though cholestasis may be slow to improve. Rashes, fever, joint pain and eosinophilia may provide evidence of an allergic process. Liver biopsy is often inconclusive. The drugs below are commoner offenders.

Antibiotics	— Isoniazid, pyrazinamide, rifampicin, PAS, sulphonamides, nitrofurantoin, erythromycin estolate.
Anaesthetics	— halothane.
Antidepressants	— tricyclics and monoamine oxidase inhibitors.
Antineoplastic agents	— azathioprine.
Antirheumatics	— phenylbutazone, penicillamine, gold.
Antidiabetics	— tolbutamide, chlorpropamide.
Anticonvulsants	— phenytoin, sodium valproate.
Antihypertensives	— methyldopa.
Anxiolytics	— phenothiazines.

Chapter Seventeen

HEART DISEASE

The standard chest radiograph and electrocardiogram are the basic investigative techniques in cardiac problems and are sufficient for most patients. Specialized invasive investigations are usually performed only if surgery is contemplated. They include angiography of either the left or right side of the heart, combined with measurements of pressure and oxygen saturation and coronary arteriography.

Specialized non-invasive investigation is of increasing importance and is gradually reducing the need for invasive tests. It includes echocardiography, exercise tests, phonocardiography and apexcardiography. Isotope methods are also used to study myocardial perfusion, left-to-right shunts and ventricular function. Myocardial imaging with thallium-201 is a sensitive method of detecting regional myocardial ischaemia.

Radiology
The standard posteroanterior view (PA) taken with the cassette at 6 ft (1.8 m) from the tube target gives information about the size of the heart chambers, the aorta, pulmonary trunk and main pulmonary vessels. Pulmonary plethora and left heart failure are shown. Anteroposterior views taken in ill patients exaggerate the size of the heart because it is further from the cassette. Supine views may wrongly suggest pulmonary vein congestion.

Cineradiography of the heart can be used to study pulsation of the chambers.

Electrocardiography — see Chapter 18.

Echocardiography
The image produced by ultrasound (p. 9) reflected from cardiac structures is recorded on paper. A single beam (M-mode) is often

used. The impulse rate is 1000 per second, so a kind of one-dimensional moving picture is obtained. Two-dimensional (real-time) pictures can be obtained by using multiple beams or a scanner. They are easier to interpret and superior for some purposes, but the equipment is more expensive.

Echocardiography is the best technique for detecting pericardial fluid and thickening. Myocardial disease can be detected. It is also very useful in valvular disease. Unsuspected mitral or acute stenosis can be revealed. Organic and functional mitral incompetence can be differentiated. Vegetations may be seen on heart valves. Atrial myxomas are well shown.

CLINICAL PROBLEMS

Angina
This diagnosis is based on the patient's story and the answer to diagnostic doubt is usually a more careful history taken by a clinician conversant with the characteristics of anginal pain, as usually physical signs are absent and the ECG is normal at rest. The main differential diagnosis includes musculoskeletal pain, oesophageal pain and cardiac neurosis. Problems arise when the story is unclear and when more than one type of pain is present. Also, an abnormal ECG does not prove the pain is cardiac and an abnormal barium swallow does not prove it is oesophageal. Relevant tests include exercise electrocardiography and isotope imaging, echocardiography, examination of the oesophagus, therapeutic tests, and coronary angiography.

Exercise electrocardiogram
If the ECG is normal, the patient is exercised under medical supervision and the ECG is repeated. Pain with an abnormal ECG favours angina, whereas if the ECG remains normal, other aetiology should be considered. An abnormal ECG without pain may indicate the presence of ischaemic heart disease, a common finding, but it does not prove that the pain is cardiac in origin. Observation of the patient is itself informative. Like all provocative tests it can be dangerous. Trinitrate tablets should be available and resuscitative equipment should be within call. Various techniques and criteria of abnormality are used. ST-segment depression in the standard and lateral leads is sought. Flat or downward sloping segments are more

significant than upward sloping ones. Depression has to be more than 1 mm to be significant. The test is more reliable in men than women.

Other tests
Myocardium which becomes ischaemic during exertion can be demonstrated by a thallium isotope. Echocardiography can demonstrate cardiomyopathy and valvular disease. Both angina and oesophagitis may appear to respond to bicarbonate or glyceryl trinitrate, but propranolol is specific for the former and cimetidine for the latter.

Acute Myocardial Infarction
In the evaluation of suspected myocardial infarction confirmatory evidence is sought and other diagnoses are considered. These include pulmonary embolism, spontaneous pneumothorax, dissecting aneurysm, pericarditis, oesophageal and spinal pain, and upper abdominal problems. Most help is obtained from the ECG, chest X-ray and serum enzymes. If infarction cannot be confirmed, the diagnosis may be wrong—the pain may represent coronary insufficiency rather than infarction, or the infarction may be small.

ECG (Fig. 17.1)
Abnormalities of the Q and T waves and the ST segment are seen. Acute infarction cannot be definitely diagnosed from the cardiogram alone if only one of these is abnormal. Serial recordings are very helpful. Changes due to previous infarction, pericarditis and pulmonary embolism can mislead.

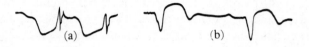

Figure 17.1 Acute myocardial infarction, lead V3. (a) Early. (b) Approximately one week later.

1. ST segment. This changes first. Initially it is elevated straight or slightly concave upwards, merging with a tall T wave. Later it is convex upwards and the T wave gradually inverts. Leads opposite undamaged myocardium show ST segment depression.

2. Q wave—pathological Q waves appear and may persist (p. 184).
3. The T wave is initially tall, and then deep, symmetrical T-wave inversion appears and may persist.

Enzymes

These should be taken as soon as possible and repeated on two successive mornings if there is any clinical doubt. The extent and duration of the enzyme elevation is roughly proportional to the size of the infarction. The AST rise is higher than the ALT rise unless there is also pulmonary embolism or liver congestion. If enzyme elevation is associated with cardiac pain, infarction is probable even in the absence of ECG evidence.

Table 17.1 Enzyme rises after myocardial infarction

	First possible rise (h)	Peak (h)	Maximum duration rise (days)
Creatine phosphokinase	3	24	3
Aspartate aminotransferase	6	36	6
Lactate dehydrogenase	12	60	12

Other evidence

A polymorphonuclear leucocytosis can start by 12 hours, the ESR may rise and pyrexia may start on the second day. Left ventricular failure may be seen on the CXR.

Pulmonary Embolism

Small emboli to the lung periphery usually cause symptoms when they give rise to infarction. Tachypnoea, haemoptysis and evidence of pleurisy are typical but not invariable. Central pulmonary emboli occluding a major artery cause marked tachypnoea, collapse and cyanosis. They are often preceded by small emboli. Chronic thromboembolic pulmonary hypertension is a rare cause of unexplained dyspnoea. Obvious peripheral vein thrombosis is often absent.

ECG

Abnormalities are frequent but often non-specific and transient. Common findings are T-wave inversion in V1–3, right-axis deviation and the S_1,Q_3,T_3 pattern (prominent S in I and a Q and inverted T in III). Right bundle branch block also occurs.

Imaging
Chest X-ray is necessary to exclude other pathology and it may show changes suspicious of infarction, with wedge-shaped consolidation pointing medially. The signs of oligaemia due to major embolism without infarction are subtle.

Combined ventilation and perfusion isotope scans are helpful. Typically, perfusion is absent from areas where ventilation is normal and the X-ray shows no changes.

Pulmonary angiography is indicated where surgery is considered for major embolism. As most emboli come from the leg veins, bilateral normal venograms provide evidence against embolism.

Other tests
Pyrexia and leucocytosis occur with infarction as with pneumonia, but the leucocytosis is moderate and there is no left shift unless infection supervenes. The sputum is usually mixed bloody and mucoid, but not purulent until infection supervenes. Pleural effusions are often haemorrhagic but not always. The serum bilirubin and enzymes may rise, but this is not specific. A low arterial PO_2 and PCO_2 is a combination typical of major pulmonary embolism. Fibrin degeneration products often appear in the circulation.

Hypertension
Investigation assesses three aspects: the damage already caused by hypertension, its cause, and other causes of arterial damage. It is generally more profitable to study total management of the hypertensive rather than to seek rare causes. Increased risk is seen with males, and if cigarette smoking, high serum cholesterol level, diabetes or an abnormal ECG are found.

Hypertensive damage
Investigation centres on a search for evidence of left ventricular damage (CXR, ECG) and renal damage (serum creatinine, urine protein).

Primary causes of hypertension

These are sought mainly in the young severe hypertensive, e.g. under 40 with a diastolic pressure of 120 mm Hg or more. Failure to respond to treatment, a clinical clue, or absence of a family history might also indicate a search.

1. Drugs—contraceptive pill, liquorice.
2. Renal disease—renal artery stenosis, renal parenchymal disease.
3. Adrenal disease—Conn's syndrome, phaeochromocytoma, Cushing's syndrome.
4. Coarctation of the aorta.

Tests

In hospital practice the following are reasonable screening tests before starting treatment:

1. Full blood count and ESR—for polycythaemia and arteritis.
2. Urinalysis and urine deposit—for renal disease and secondary renal damage.
3. Serum urea and electrolytes (before starting diuretics)—for hyperaldosteronism and renal damage.
4. CXR and ECG—for evidence of left ventricular damage and coarctation.
5. Cholesterol and blood sugar—for other risk factors.
6. Special tests—IVU and renography are indicated in a young severe hypertensive or if there is a suggestion of renal arterial or parenchymal damage. Renal biopsy, renal angiography or renin levels may be appropriate.

Valvular Disease

The preliminary diagnosis is clinical. Plain X-ray of the chest gives information about valvular calcification, the size of the heart chambers and the pulmonary circulation. Echocardiography supplements this and enables direct study of valve movement. Angiography and the study of pressure and oxygen saturation in the cardiac chambers is usually needed only when surgery is contemplated.

The commonest cause of valvular disease in adults is still rheumatic heart disease. Congenital conditions must also be considered. Mitral valve insufficiency may be caused by endocarditis or ischaemic papillary muscle dysfunction. Aortic regurgitation may be related to endocarditis, syphilitic aortitis and connective tissue disorders, such as Marfan's syndrome and ankylosing spondylitis.

Pericardial Disease

Clinical findings are supplemented by electrocardiography, radiology and echocardiography.

The cardiogram may remain normal. Often ST-segment elevation, concave upwards, appears first, followed by relatively shallow T-wave inversion. Abnormal Q waves and reciprocal ST-segment depression, which occur with infarction, do not appear. With effusions, the limb leads may show low voltage.

Radiological enlargement of the cardiac silhouette may be due to effusion or dilatation of the chambers, but the echocardiogram can demonstrate effusions even below 100 ml by a characteristic echo-free area. Pericardial aspiration may be necessary to determine the cause of an effusion.

The differentiation of a primary pericarditis from pericarditis due to acute myocardial infarction may be difficult as enzyme changes and arrhythmias can occur in pericarditis. In acute pericarditis the fever and rub occur on the first day and the cardiographic findings differ, as above.

Cor Pulmonale

Acute cor pulmonale most often follows massive pulmonary embolism (p. 173) and also occurs in fat embolism. Chronic cor pulmonale is most usually due to obstructive airways disease, but occurs with any chronic lung disease.

The venous pressure is always high. The cardiogram usually shows signs of right atrial or ventricular enlargement (p. 197). The chest X-ray shows an enlarged pulmonary trunk and main pulmonary artery branches, with oligaemia of the peripheral lung fields. There is hypoxaemia and hypercapnia.

Cardiomyopathy

In congestive cardiomyopathy there is dilatation of the ventricles and heart failure without much hypertrophy. Organic valvular disease, hypertension and ischaemic heart disease must be excluded. There are several causes, which include alcoholism and thyroid disease.

Hypertrophic cardiomyopathy may resemble aortic stenosis clinically. The echocardiogram demonstrates marked thickening of the ventricular septum. Restrictive cardiomyopathy and constrictive pericarditis which has not caused radiological calcification may be difficult to diagnose. Study of jugular pulse tracings and cardiac catheterization may be necessary. Constrictive pericarditis must be considered when right heart failure is neither due to cor pulmonale, nor secondary to left heart failure, or when cirrhosis of the liver is associated with high pressures in the jugular veins.

Chapter Eighteen

ELECTROCARDIOGRAPHY

INTRODUCTION

Lead Positions

The standard bipolar leads of the electrocardiogram I, II and III and the unipolar limb leads AVR, AVL, and AVF 'look' at the heart in the frontal or coronal plane (Fig. 18.1). The six chest leads V1 to V6 are in the horizontal plane (Fig. 18.2). V1 is taken in the fourth intercostal space at the right sternal border, V2 in the fourth space at

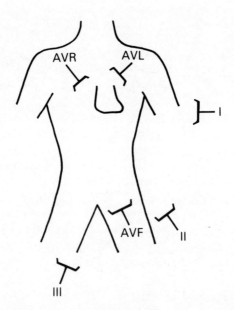

Figure 18.1   Coronal section of the body, showing the bipolar and unipolar limb leads.

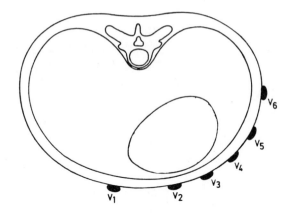

Figure 18.2 Transverse section of the body, showing the chest leads.

the left border, V3 between V2 and V4, V4 in the fifth space in the midclavicular line and V5 and V6 in the fifth space in the anterior and mid-axillary lines respectively. In the normal heart leads I, AVL and V5–7 'look' at the left ventricle, V2 at the septum and V1 at the right ventricle. Leads III and AVF 'look' at the inferior surface of the heart.

Complex Intervals and Duration
In the standard electrocardiogram (Fig. 18.3), one small square = 1 mm = 0.04 sec at the standard writer speed (25 mm/sec) and one large square = 5 mm = 0.2 sec. The gap between complexes (R–R interval) gives the ventricular rate.

The gap between the atrial (P) and the ventricular (QRS) complexes and the duration of the QRS complex give information about the conducting system of the heart. The duration of the P wave is increased in left atrial hypertrophy and the duration of the R wave is increased in left ventricular hypertrophy.

Complex Height and Direction
The graph paper of the electrocardiogram is calibrated so that 10 mm = 1 mV. When the electrical impulse flows towards an electrode, a positive or upward deflection of the tracing is recorded,

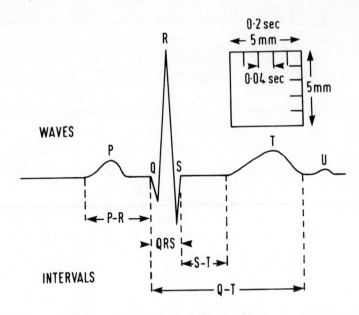

Figure 18.3 ECG complex.

and when it flows away, a negative deflection is recorded. As the left ventricle is the dominant chamber of the heart, i.e. contains the most muscle, leads facing the left ventricle are normally positive and leads facing the right ventricle are normally negative. The height of the deflections is increased by hypertrophy of muscle but also when the chest wall is thin. The height of the waves and elevation of the segments is measured from the top of the baseline to the top of the segment or wave. Depressions are measured from the bottom of lines. In some conventions complexes smaller than 5 mm are written with a small letter and larger ones with a capital letter, e.g. qR.

Analysis of the Electrocardiogram

When examining a tracing (Fig. 18.4), the heart rate is determined from the duration of the R–R interval. The rhythm is determined from the regularity and duration of the R–R interval and the relationship between the P waves and the QRS complex. The sizes of the complexes in the different leads are compared to determine the cardiac axis (Fig. 18.21). The P wave, the QRS complex, the ST segment and the T wave are studied to assess the state of the myocardium and the conducting system.

WAVES AND INTERVALS (Fig. 18.3)

P Wave
Atrial depolarization; usually best studied in II and VI.

Height
Not more than 2.5 mm (3mm in I, II, III); increased in right atrial enlargement (Fig. 18.5), when it is usually peaked in shape.

Duration
Less than 0.12 sec; increased and often notched in left atrial enlargement (Fig. 18.6). (Best seen in I, V1 and V5).

Direction
Upright in I, II, AVF, V3–6, inverted in AVR, in either direction or biphasic in III and V1–2. In ectopic atrial activation P is typically upright in AVR and inverted in AVF, but there may only be a slight change in waveform if the ectopic focus is near the sinus node. P waves are absent in atrial fibrillation (p. 192), sinoatrial block and may be unrecognizable in escape rhythms and tachycardias.

P–R Interval
Atrioventricular conduction time. Beginning of P wave to beginning of QRS complex. Normally not more than 0.20 s in adults and 0.18 s in children. Tachycardia reduces the interval and the upper limit of normal is then less. An increase is first-degree heart block (see Fig. 18.16), which is seen with myocardial ischaemia, rheumatic fever and digitalis.

A short PR interval (below 0.10 s) is sometimes seen in nodal rhythm and is usual in Wolff–Parkinson–White syndrome.

QRS Complex
Ventricular depolarization. The Q wave is the negative deflection preceding an R wave. The R wave is the first positive deflection and the S wave is the negative deflection after the R wave. R^1 is a further positive wave after the S wave. A QS complex occurs when there is

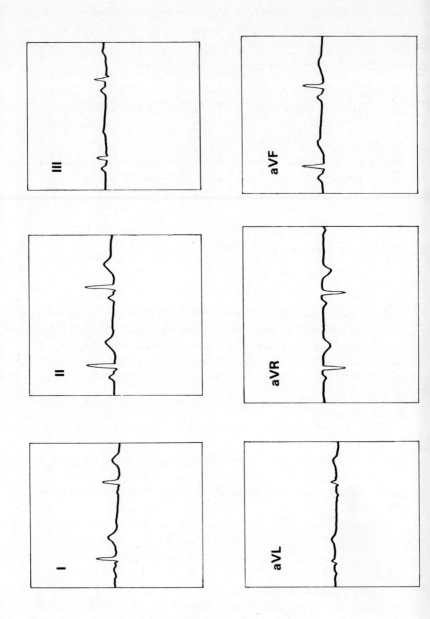

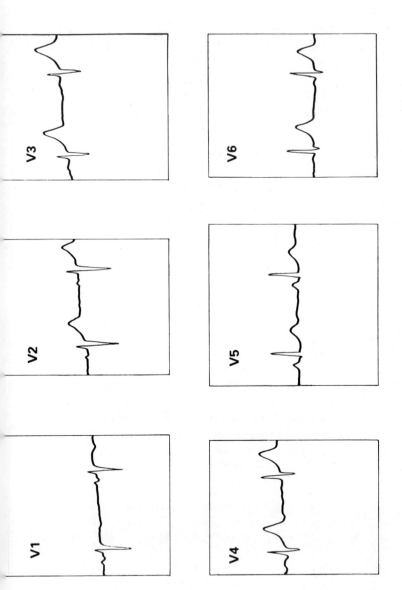

Figure 18.4 Normal electrocardiogram. Rate 70/min; rhythm sinus; Axis +60.

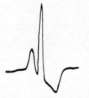

Figure 18.5 Right atrial hypertrophy, lead II.

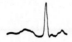

Figure 18.6 Left atrial hypertrophy, lead II.

no R wave. The normal duration is 0.05–0.10 s. Increased duration is seen in bundle branch block and hyperkalaemia.

Q Wave

A normal Q wave lasts less than 0.04 s. and is less than 4 mm deep or less than 25% of the following R wave. Deep Q waves or QS complexes are normal in AVR and V1. Pathological Q waves occur in:

1. Myocardial infarction—recent and old, the commonest cause.
2. Left ventricular hypertrophy (V5–6).
3. Right ventricular hypertrophy (V1–4, II, III, AVF).
4. Left bundle branch block (V1–4).
5. Emphysema (II, III, AVF).

These conditions are distinguished by their other characteristics. A single abnormal Q wave is not always significant. Q waves in III are not significant if there are no abnormal Q waves in II and AVF.

QT Interval

The duration of electrical systole measured from the onset of the QRS complex wave to the end of the T wave. Normally about 0.43 s. and reducing by roughly 0.05 s. for every 20 beats above 60/min. At usual rates it is not more than half the R–R interval.

Prolongation
1. Myocardial disease—infarction, myopathy, myocarditis.
2. Drugs—procainamide, quinidine.
3. Hypocalcaemia.

Shortening is seen in hypercalcaemia and with digitalis.

ST Segment
Its position is compared with the TP segment.

Elevation
Normally up to 3 mm in V1–3 and 1 mm in other leads, but sometimes greater in Africans. Abnormal in:
1. Myocardial infarction—convex upwards.
2. Pericarditis—concave upwards.
3. Angina—only in the Prinzmetal variety.
4. Ventricular aneurysm—the elevation is persistent.

Depression
Normally not more than 0.5 mm in all leads except AVR (and AVL in right axis deviation). An upward sloping depression may be seen in sinus tachycardia. Abnormal in:
1. Myocardial ischaemia—especially in II, V5–6. A flat or downward sloping depression is most significant.
2. Myocardial infarction—either local or subendocardial, or reciprocal to ST elevation elsewhere.
3. Left ventricular hypertrophy (V5–6). (See Fig. 18.22.)
4. Left bundle branch block (V5–6). (See Fig. 18.20.)
5. Right ventricular failure (V1–3). It is convex upwards.
6. Right bundle branch block (V1–3). (See Fig. 18.19.)
7. Digitalis (V5–6). It slopes down with a sharp terminal rise like a reversed tick.

T Wave
Ventricular repolarization. It is at least one-tenth of the height of the R wave, but usually not more than 13 mm except in young males. It is inverted in AVR and may be in AVL, AVF, III, V1 and V2 if QRS is negative in these leads, as it points in the direction of the QRS.

Tall waves
1. Hyperkalaemia.

2. Myocardial infarction—true posterior (V1–4), recovering inferior and subendocardial.

Inversion and depression
1. Deep symmetrical—ischaemia and infarction. (Fig. 18.7).
2. Shallow—usually pathological, but non-specific.
3. Flattening—this may be pathological, but is unreliable and non-specific.

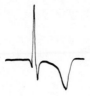

Figure 18.7   Ischaemic T-wave inversion, lead V4.

RATE AND RHYTHM

Heart Rate
To determine the ventricular rate count the number of large squares in an R–R interval (cardiac cycle) and divide it into 300. If the rate is not regular, count the number of R–R intervals in 15 large squares (3 s.) and multiply by 20. If the atrial rate differs from the ventricular rate, the same procedure is carried out with the P wave. Special rulers are available to avoid the need for calculation.

Heart Rhythm
The heart is normally activated from the sinoatrial node in the right atrium. The impulse spreads through the atria to the atrioventricular node, then down the bundle of His which splits into a right and left branch to activate the ventricles. In normal sinus rhythm a regularly occurring P wave is followed by a QRS complex. Sinus tachycardia is defined as a resting heart rate above 100/min. (above 130/min. in infants). Sinus bradycardia is a rate below 60/min. In sinus arrhythmia the P–QRS complexes are normal, but the P–P interval gradually lengthens and shortens.

Premature Impulses

These are discharges preceding the expected discharge of the prevailing rhythm. Mostly they are of ectopic origin, usually arising from the atrium or ventricle, and are called extrasystoles, though the term is not entirely accurate. Three or more occurring in succession are regarded as a tachycardia.

Supraventricular (Fig. 18.8)

Usually the QRS complex is normal and there is an abnormal P wave. If multiple, they may presage an atrial arrhythmia, but they are otherwise innocent.

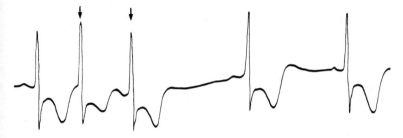

Figure 18.8   Supraventricular extrasystoles. Second and third complexes.

Ventricular (Fig. 18.9)

The QRS complex resembles a bundle branch block and there is no P wave. Heart disease is suspected in older people or if they are frequent, come in pairs, or vary in form. Digitalis toxicity and myocardial ischaemia are common causes.

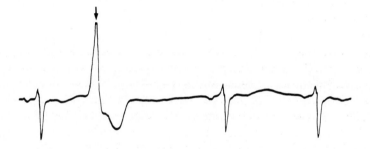

Figure 18.9   Ventricular extrasystole.

Regular Bradycardia
R–R intervals are increased but regular.

Sinus bradycardia
This occurs in myxoedema, hypothermia, obstructive jaundice, raised intracranial pressure, inferior myocardial infarction, digitalis toxicity, and normally in athletes.

Complete atrioventricular (AV) block (Fig. 18.10)
1. The P waves are not related to the QRS complex and occur regularly at a different higher rate.
2. The ventricular rate is slow, usually below 50/min.
3. The QRS complex usually has a bundle branch block pattern. It may be normal if the ventricles are activated from the bundle of His.

Advanced second-degree atrioventricular block
Alternate impulses are not conducted (2:1 block) or two or more consecutive impulses (3:1, 4:1) are not conducted.

Atrial flutter with 4:1 block (see below)

Atrioventricular junctional (nodal) rhythm
The ventricles and atria are both activated from the AV node (junction). An abnormal P wave is seen related to the QRS complex and the PR interval is shortened unless the P wave is hidden in the QRS complex. Common causes of this are acute myocardial infarction and digitalis toxicity.

Regular Tachycardia
R–R intervals are reduced but equal.

Sinus tachycardia

Supraventricular tachycardia (SVT) (Fig. 18.11)
An ectopic focus in the atrium takes over. The atrial rate is 140–240/min., often 150/min. The arrhythmia begins and ends abruptly.
1. P waves are abnormal. They may be obscured by the QRS complex. P is often upright in AVR and inverted in AVF.

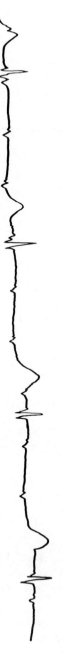

Figure 18.10 Complete heart block.

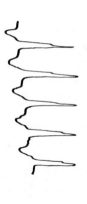

Figure 18.11 Supraventricular tachycardia, lead V1.

2. The ventricular rate is regular unless there is intermittent atrioventricular block.
3. The QRS complex is usually normal. If bundle branch block occurs the rhythm must be distinguished from ventricular tachycardia (p. 191).

Atrial flutter (Fig. 18.12)
1. Regular flutter waves with a saw-tooth appearance at about 300/min. are best seen in II.
2. Ventricular response is usually regular with 2:1 AV block, but may vary.
3. Carotid sinus massage correctly performed temporarily reduces the rate to a half or one-quarter.

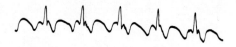

Figure 18.12   Atrial flutter, lead II.

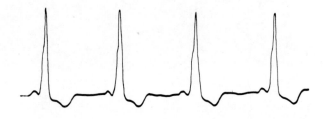

Figure 18.13   Wolff–Parkinson–White syndrome, lead II.

Wolff–Parkinson–White (WPW) Syndrome (Fig. 18.13)
There is pre-excitation of the ventricles through an extra and abnormal AV connection.
1. Short P–R interval of 0.11 s. or less.
2. Wide QRS complex of 0.11 s. or more, with slurring of the first part in some leads (delta wave).

3. Normal PJ interval of not more than 0.26 s. (J is the junction between the end of the QRS complex and the beginning of the RST segment.)
4. Right or left bundle branch block pattern, which may stimulate inferior infarction, may be seen.

WPW syndrome is associated with supraventricular tachycardia caused by circus movement of the exciting stimulus round the normal and accessory conducting bundles. Atrial fibrillation may cause a fast ventricular response and digitalis is contraindicated as it shortens the refractory period of the bypass tract.

Ventricular Tachycardia (VT) (Fig. 18.14)
An ectopic focus in the ventricle takes over.
1. P waves unrelated to QRS, but often not identified. They may follow the QRS complex but do not precede it, as may be recognized if the onset of the tachycardia is recorded.
2. QRS of bundle branch block type and wider than 0.12 s.
3. Ventricular rate slightly irregular.

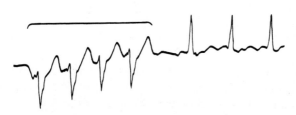

Figure 18.14 Ventricular tachycardia, lead I. Normal rhythm after four complexes.

VT must be distinguished from SVT with abnormal QRS complexes.
1. In VT the QRS complex is rarely of the right bundle branch block type, though it often is in SVT.
2. If P waves can be seen (sometimes in leads where the QRS complex is small) in VT, they are independent of and have a slower rate than the ventricles. In SVT the P waves precede the QRS complex.

3. Premature beats seen before the onset of tachycardia are similar to the tachycardia pattern in VT, but not always in SVT.
4. The patient with VT is usually ill and the arrhythmia does not respond to carotid sinus massage.

Ventricular Flutter
This life-threatening arrhythmia is similar to VT, but the QRS complexes and T waves merge into regular large or small undulations at a rate of about 250/min.

Accelerated Ventricular Rhythm (Idioventricular Tachycardia)
When the heart rate slows, e.g. after myocardial infarction or due to digitalis, a pacemaker in the AV junction or below takes over, usually at a rate below 60/min but sometimes over 100/min. The condition is benign and usually lasts less than 30 beats. Independent P wave discharges occurring slower than the ventricular rate are seen.

Irregular Rhythms
The first three below cause an irregular tachycardia.

Atrial fibrillation (Fig. 18.15)
The common causes are ischaemic heart disease, rheumatic heart disease and thyrotoxicosis. alcohol
1. First establish that the R–R interval is completely irregular.
2. Next establish the absence of definite P waves. In recent cases fibrillation waves may be seen, especially in V1.

Atrial flutter
With varying second-degree heart block.

Supraventricular tachycardia
With varying second degree heart block.

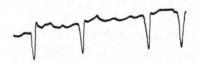

Figure 18.15   Atrial fibrillation, lead V1.

Extrasystoles
Frequent and irregular.

Sinus arrhythmia
If marked.

With bradycardia
This is seen in slow atrial fibrillation, in second-degree heart block (varying block or 3:2 or 4:3 atrial beats conducted) and in sinoatrial block where an entire PQRS complex is absent.

CONDUCTION DEFECTS

Sinoatrial Block
The sinus impulse is blocked before it reaches the atrium and the complete PQRS complex is absent.

Atrioventricular Block (AV Block)
AV block occurs in acute and chronic myocardial ischaemia and digitalis toxicity.
1. First degree (p. 181, Fig. 18.16).
2. Second degree (Fig. 18.17). Not every impulse is conducted and the frequency of conduction failure can be expressed as a ratio. In Mobitz type I (Wenckebach) block the P–R interval increases progressively until a P wave is not followed by a QRS complex (Fig. 18.18, 6:5 block). In the more serious Mobitz type II AV block the QRS complex fails to follow the P wave at regular. intervals (2:1, 3:1). The PR interval is fixed and the QRS complex is wide.
3. Third degree (complete, p. 188).

Bundle Branch Block
Conduction is blocked in one of the main branches of the bundle of His.

Right bundle branch block (RBBB) (Fig. 18.19)
1. There is a secondary R wave in V1 (imperfect M pattern).
2. S is slurred in I.
3. QRS is over 0.10 s. if the block is complete.

194

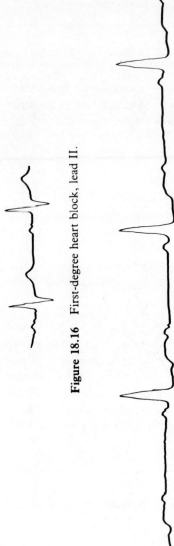

Figure 18.16 First-degree heart block, lead II.

Figure 18.17 Second-degree heart block (Mobitz type II), lead I.

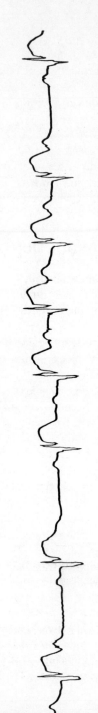

Figure 18.18 Second-degree heart block (with Wenckebach phenomenon following myocardial infarction), lead II.

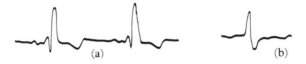

Figure 18.19   Right bundle branch block. (a) Lead V1 (b) Lead I.

4. T wave inversion in right precordial leads.

RBBB may be normal, or associated with ischaemic heart disease (it does not mask q waves), right ventricular hypertrophy, atrial septal defect or pulmonary embolism.

Left bundle branch block (LBBB) (Fig. 18.20)
1. A secondary R wave (imperfect M) complex in V6 with no q waves.
2. A wide QS complex in right ventricular leads.
3. QRS is over 0.11 s if the block is complete.
4. T wave inversion in left precordial leads.

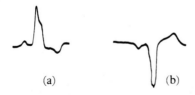

Figure 18.20   Left bundle branch block. (a) Lead V6 (b) Lead V1.

LBBB usually results from acute or chronic ischaemic heart disease. It obscures the signs of acute myocardial infarction, which cannot be diagnosed by the electrocardiogram in its presence.

Fascicular blocks (hemiblocks)
The left bundle divides into two branches or fascicles. Interruption of either changes the QRS axis without widening the QRS complex considerably. In anterior fascicular block the QRS complex is more negative than −45°. In lead II it is predominantly negative. Posterior

block is rare and is usually associated with RBBB. The QRS axis is +120° or more in the absence of the usual causes of right axis deviation.

CARDIAC AXIS

The predominant direction of the electrical forces of the heart is the cardiac axis. The axis may be determined for the P and T waves and QRS complex in the frontal, sagittal or horizontal plane, but only the axis of the QRS complex in the frontal and horizontal plane is discussed. It depends on the anatomical position of the heart and the direction of depolarization through the ventricles.

Determination of Frontal Plane Axis (Fig. 18.21)

Normal
−15° to +90°

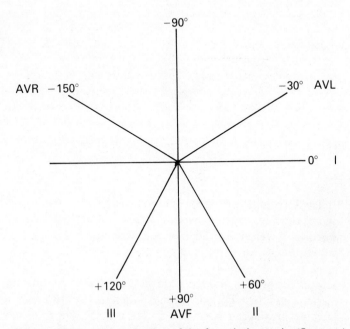

Figure 18.21 Determination of the frontal plane axis. (See text.)

From the limb leads (Fig. 18.1), rotation of the heart round an axis from sternum to spine is determined. The axis will point towards the most positive lead, and in the lead at right angles to the axis the sum of the negative and positive QRS deflections will most nearly equal zero. If the latter lead is slightly negative the axis points 105° away from it, but if it is slightly positive the axis only points 75° away.

Right axis deviation (axis more positive than +90°)
Usually lead III is tall and taller than lead II and lead I is predominantly negative. This may be normal but it is seen in right ventricular hypertrophy and emphysema. A rightward shift may occur in acute pulmonary embolism.

Left axis deviation (axis more negative than −15°)
Lead AVL is tall and lead II is negative. This can be seen in left anterior fascicular block and left ventricular hypertrophy, but can be normal.

Horizontal Plane Rotation
This takes place round an axis from head to foot and it is clockwise or counter-clockwise looking up from below. Diagnosis is from the precordial leads. The normal transition from right ventricular rS to left ventricular qR occurs with an RS complex in V4.

Clockwise rotation—the right ventricle faces anteriorly and V1–6 leads record rS complexes; the left ventricular qR complex only appears in V6. This occurs with right ventricular hypertrophy and pulmonary embolism, but it may also be seen in normals.

Counter-clockwise rotation—the left ventricle rotates to the front and left ventricular qR complexes appear in V4 and even in V3. This occurs with left ventricular hypertrophy.

VENTRICULAR HYPERTROPHY

To make the diagnosis all clinical, cardiographic and radiological evidence must be summated.

Right Ventricular Hypertrophy
1. Dominant R waves in right ventricular leads: R is at least 5 mm tall and larger than S in V1.
2. Right axis deviation and clockwise rotation.

3. T wave inversion in right ventricular leads.
4. Right bundle branch block—partial or complete.
It occurs in pulmonary disease, mitral stenosis and congenital heart disease, and acutely in pulmonary embolism.

Left Ventricular Hypertrophy (Fig. 18.22)
1. Counter-clockwise rotation and left axis deviation.
2. Tall R waves in I, V4–6 and AVL, with deep S waves in V1–2, R in V5 + S in V2 greater than 35 mm.
3. Increased duration of the QRS complex.
4. Slight ST segment depression with broadly inverted T waves over left ventricular leads.

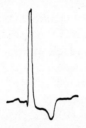

Figure 18.22   Left ventricular hypertrophy, lead V6.

Myocardial Infarction
See Chapter 17.

Drugs and Electrolytes

Potassium
The first sign of hyperkalaemia is tall, peaked T waves. The PR interval prolongs and the QRS complex widens until a large undulating sine wave appears before the onset of asystole. Hypokalaemia causes ST segment depression and flattening or shallow inversion of the T wave, followed by a prominent U wave.

Calcium
Hypercalcaemia shortens and hypocalcaemia lengthens the QT interval.

Digitalis
Properly digitalized patients may show a shallow, concave upwards, scooped ST segment depression. Toxicity causes ventricular extrasystoles, arrhythmias and conduction defects.

Other drugs
Quinidine, procainamide and disopyramide prolong the QT interval, flatten the T wave and produce U waves. Phenothiazine drugs may have a similar effect.

Specialized Electrocardiographic Tests
Exercise electrocardiography is discussed in Chapter 18. Ambulatory (Holter) electrocardiography is useful in the assessment of recurrent arrhythmias, syncope which might be of cardiac origin and other symptoms which might be related to disorders or cardiac rhythm. The tracing may be recorded after hyperventilation for 30 s recumbent and repeated on standing. T-wave inversion in the inferior and lateral leads may be shown to mimic myocardial ischaemia by this means.

Physiological Variations
Infants have a pattern of right ventricular hypertrophy with tall R waves until aged 5 and inverted T waves in the right precordial leads until aged 10. The cardiac axis points to the right in children. The PR interval is shorter (p. 181).

In pregnancy, the axis shifts to the left by about 15°. T is flat or negative in III. A q wave appears in III and AVF. In Africans, T-wave inversion may persist in right-sided leads until the third decade. ST segment elevation up to 4 mm may be seen in left precordial leads in young adults.

With age the cardiac axis becomes more negative.

Chapter Nineteen

CHEST DISEASE

IMAGING

Radiology

The posteroanterior X-ray taken at 1.8 m is the basic investigation. Anteroposterior views, necessary in ill patients, exaggerate the size of the heart. A lateral film is necessary to determine the precise anatomical site of a lesion. Penetrated views may better define lesions obscured by other structures. Lordotic views are helpful for apical lesions. Tomography enables better definition of solid lesions. Computerized tomography (CT) can demonstrate metastases not otherwise shown and is useful in the study of mediastinal lesions. Bronchography may be used for the assessment of bronchiectasis and selective bronchography through the bronchoscope can be used to locate the source of haemoptysis.

Isotope Studies

Ventilation can be studied with radioactive xenon and perfusion with technetium-labelled albumin. Combined studies are useful in pulmonary embolism (p. 173) and obstructive airways disease.

Ultrasound

This is useful in pleural disease. Fluid can be correctly located and distinguished from a solid lesion.

Bronchoscopy

Fibreoptic bronchoscopes have increased the scope of bronchoscopy because of their safety and convenience. Transbronchial biopsy, transbronchial needle aspiration, bronchial brushings and bronchoalveolar lavage are techniques which can provide cells or tissue for study. Selective bronchography is also possible. By the appropriate bronchoscopic technique it may be possible to diagnose discrete lesions such as carcinomas and mediastinal lymph nodes and diffuse diseases such as sarcoidosis and cryptogenic fibrosing alveolitis.

SECRETIONS

Sputum

It is necessary to obtain an adequate specimen from the lower respiratory tract, preferably in the early morning. Inspection of this specimen is the most reliable guide to the presence of infection. A purulent sputum indicates infection, whereas a colourless mucoid appearance is good evidence against it. Exceptions occur to most rules and the sputum may appear mucoid in tuberculosis or may be green owing to eosinophilia.

Sputum microscopy

Moderate numbers of all forms of bacteria, usually normal mouth flora, are seen, but large numbers of a single organism may indicate a relevant pathogen. Gram-positive diplococci suggest a pneumococcal infection, whereas clusters of Gram-positive cocci are probably staphylococci and Gram-negative pleomorphic cocco-bacilli are probably *Haemophilus influenzae*. Gram-negative bacilli may be just contaminants or may represent a pseudomonas or 'coliform' infection in a debilitated patient. A rapid provisional identification of a possible pathogen may thus be made sometimes even when it later fails to grow in culture because of previous antibiotic treatment.

Polymorphonuclear leucocytes occur with infection. Staining for eosinophils may reveal an allergic factor. When a bronchial carcinoma is suspected serial samples are examined for malignant cells.

Sputum culture

In exacerbations of chronic bronchitis infection is usually due to pneumococci and *H. influenzae*. A culture should be requested if there is no response to treatment. Accurate microbiological diagnosis is very important with pneumonia. Specimens of sputum, blood and pleural fluid, if obtainable, should be cultured. A physiotherapist may be helpful in obtaining a sputum specimen. As always, the suspected diagnosis must be indicated to the bacteriologist. Tubercle bacilli, anaerobic organisms and fungi require special culture techniques.

Str. viridans and *N. catarrhalis* are commensals. *C. albicans* occurs commonly after antibiotic treatment but rarely invades the bronchi. Pneumococci and staphylococci can be commensals but must be assumed to be pathogens in the presence of pneumonia. *H. influenzae* is the commonest Gram-negative pathogen but *Klebsiella pneumoniae* causes cavitating pneumonia. Other Gram-negative organisms cause pneumonia in debilitated patients.

Pleural Fluid
Where pleural effusion has no obvious cause a laboratory investigation of the fluid is indicated. Most fluids are straw-coloured whatever the pathology. Chest X-ray before and after aspiration may reveal neoplastic or tuberculous lesions. A paradoxical mediastinal shift towards the effusion suggests lung collapse due to possible malignancy. Pleural biopsy with the Abrams punch is most helpful in the diagnosis of tuberculosis and malignancy. It is sometimes coupled routinely with aspiration.

Cells
1. Red cells—large numbers on microscopy or obviously bloody fluid are found with pulmonary infarction and with malignancy and rarely tuberculosis. If the tap has been traumatic, blood clears as the fluid is withdrawn.
2. Polymorphonuclear cells—these predominate in empyema, post-pneumonic sterile effusion and in association with subphrenic infection. They may also do so with pulmonary infarction, carcinoma and rarely in early tuberculosis.
3. Lymphocytes—these predominate in tuberculosis and malignancy.
4. Eosinophils—marked eosinophilia may be found, but it is often not diagnostically helpful except in that it is unusual in tuberculosis or malignancy.
5. Malignant cells—false-positives can occur, especially after pulmonary infarction and the appearances are difficult to interpret. A positive report by a skilled cytologist is of great value.
6. Mesothelial cells—these are common in malignancy and pulmonary infarction, but not in tuberculosis.

Bacteriology
Gram stain, culture and staining and culture for tubercle bacilli must always be done. Anaerobic culture is necessary in empyema.

Biochemistry
Exudates have a protein content of over 25 g/l and occur with local inflammation and increased capillary permeability. Transudates have a lower protein concentration and are caused by an increase in hydrostatic pressure in capillaries or lymphatics, or a reduction in plasma oncotic pressure. They occur in cardiac failure, hypoproteinaemia and lymphatic obstruction by neoplasm. The protein concentration of effusions is, however, often borderline.

Exudates usually have a lactate dehydrogenase (LDH) level of over 550 IU/l, and LDH levels may be especially high in malignancy and rheumatoid disease. Glucose concentrations may be below 2.0 mmol/l in empyema, malignancy and rheumatoid disease. A high cholesterol level occurs in any chronic effusion.

Causes of effusion
1. Malignancy—typically bloody and recurrent after aspiration, but often straw coloured: lymphocytes and mesothelial cells are common. Cytology or pleural biopsy may be positive. A high LDH in a transudate is suggestive.
2. Post-pneumonic—a clear or turbid but not bloody fluid containing neutrophil polymorphs. It usually starts during treatment for pneumonia and culture is negative.
3. Infarction—haemorrhagic or straw coloured, pleomorphic often with eosinophils. A lung scan after aspiration may be helpful.
4. Tuberculosis—typically a straw coloured lymphocytic exudate with negative bacteriology and a positive Mantoux test in a younger person. Pleural biopsy is often positive, but culture is not.
5. Abdominal inflammation—a usually left-sided polymorphonuclear exudate. The amylase may be high in pancreatitis and oesophageal rupture.
6. Rheumatoid disease—an exudate with a low glucose level, high LDH and positive rheumatoid factor. In SLE, antinuclear factor may be present and complement may be low.

7. Empyema—a thick, purulent fluid with more than 100 000 cells/ml. Gram stain, aerobic or anaerobic culture are usually positive.

PULMONARY FUNCTION TESTS (PFT)

The following tests of lung function are in common use:
1. Lung volumes—total lung capacity (TLC), residual volume (RV), vital capacity (VC).
2. Air flow—forced vital capacity (FVC), forced expiratory volume in one second (FEV_1), peak expiratory flow rate (PEFR).
3. Gas transfer—carbon monoxide transfer test.
4. Blood gases—PCO_2, PO_2.

Of these, the most useful and widely available are measurements of air flow and blood gases. Several of the tests require co-operation from the patient, so practice runs are necessary. Normal values are derived from tables which adjust for height, age and sex, and abnormality is definite only where the result is 20% different from that predicted. The tests are more useful in assessing the severity of disease and its response to treatment than in diagnosis.

Lung Volumes
They are often measured by helium dilution methods. Total lung capacity is high in emphysema and asthma and low in diffuse pulmonary fibrosis. Residual volume is high in all forms of obstructive airways disease but may be reduced in restrictive disease.

Vital capacity
Air is expired slowly after a maximal inspiration and normally it is slightly less than the forced vital capacity, but in severe emphysema, usually clinically obvious, it may be slightly greater. It is useful in monitoring the progress and response to treatment of restrictive lung disease and also of respiratory failure due to neuromuscular disease.

Air-Flow Tests
These usually utilize portable spirometers which measure the volume and velocity of expired air.

Forced vital capacity (FVC)
Approximate normal values (litres):

Adult males	Height (cm) $\div$ 35
Adult females	Height (cm) $\div$ 43
Children	Age (yrs) $\div$ 4.5

This is the quantity of air exhaled in a single forced expiration following a maximal inspiration. It is reduced in most forms of cardiorespiratory disease.

Forced expiratory volume (FEV_1)

This is the quantity of air exhaled in the first second of a forced expiration. It falls with any reduction in FVC and the ratio FEV_1/FVC should be calculated to assess airways obstruction. At age 20 it should be over 80% and at age 60 over 70%. The FEV_1 itself is useful for monitoring disease.

Peak expiratory flow rate $(PEFR_1, PFR)$

Normal		
Adult male	over 550 l/min.	variation with age and height.
Adult female	over 400 l/min.	
Children	95 l/min. at 0.9 m and increasing by about 6 l/min/cm height.	

This is the maximum flow rate over 10 ms at the beginning of a forced expiration. A fall is slightly more specific for airways obstruction than is a fall in FEV_1.

Gas Transfer

The transfer factor for carbon monoxide (TLCO) provides a non-specific test of the gas-exchanging function of the lung. If a weak concentration of carbon monoxide (CO) is inhaled the quantity passing from the alveoli to the pulmonary capillary blood can be calculated from the CO concentration in exhaled air. Usually a steady-state method is used, but there is a single breath method, which is more sensitive, though less reliable. It is affected by several factors, including the total alveolar area and the matching of ventilation and perfusion. Reduced transfer occurs with pulmonary infiltration, emphysema and vascular occlusion and may be associated with hypoxia, especially on exertion. Rarely the test is abnormal when CXR and all other PFT are normal, so it is considered in unexplained dyspnoea and early industrial lung disease. Apparent increased transfer may occur when there is blood in the alveoli.

Blood Gases

An arterial specimen should be taken into a heparin moistened syringe and the syringe capped to seal off the blood. The specimen is put on ice and the estimation performed within an hour, even sooner if a plastic rather than a glass syringe is used. Arterialized capillary blood is less reliable but more convenient in children. Falsely high P_{CO_2} and falsely low P_{O_2} and pH readings may be obtained.

The brachial artery or the radial artery of the non-dominant side is used. An ulnar artery should be present in the latter case. Blood must be seen to pulsate in the syringe. The puncture area should be first anaesthetized and firm pressure is necessary after withdrawal of the needle.

P_{CO_2} is a good index of alveolar ventilation not much affected by ventilation/perfusion mismatching. P_{O_2} reflects the efficiency of gas exchange.

CO$_2$ Tension (P_{CO_2})

Normal (arterial)

Adult male	4.7–6.4 kPa
Adult female	4.3–6.0 kPa
Neonates	3.6–5.3 kPa
Infants	3.6–5.5 kPa
Pregnancy	a slight reduction occurs.

Increase (hypercapnia)
1. Lung disease—obstructive airways disease, classically chronic bronchitis, is the commonest cause of hypoventilation, but it may occur in any severe lung disease. In asthma the P_{CO_2} may initially fall, but in more severe attacks it rises and this is a dangerous sign.
2. Respiratory centre depression—sedatives, oxygen treatment (see below), intracranial disease.
3. Miscellaneous—obesity (Pickwickian syndrome), peripheral neuropathy.
4. Metabolic alkalosis (p. 41).

Decrease (hypocapnia)
This is due to hyperventilation. Alkalosis may result. A respiratory alkalosis may be produced by the stress of arterial puncture.
1. Respiratory disease—diffusion defects such as infiltrations, fibrosis, and oedema; unilateral lung defects, e.g. pneumonia; mild and moderate asthma.
2. Cardiovascular—pulmonary embolism and left ventricular failure.
3. Metabolic acidosis.
4. Miscellaneous—voluntary hyperventilation, cerebral damage, pyrexia, heat stroke, mechanical ventilation and anaesthesia, hepatic coma, and hypoxia due to altitude.

Effects of changes
Hypercapnia can cause headache, drowsiness and peripheral vasodilation, then twitching, papilloedema and finally coma. Symptoms appear at levels of over 8 kPa, though not always in chronic cases, and coma is usual at levels of over 16 kPa. Hypocapnia causes cerebral vasoconstriction, alkalosis, paraesthesiae, tetany and syncope.

Oxygen Tension (Po_2)

Normal (arterial)
10.6–13.3 kPa

Decrease (hypoxia)
1. With a raised Pco_2—the commonest cause is ventilatory failure due to obstructive airways disease. Oxygen must be given with caution here because removal of the hypoxic drive to respiration may cause dangerous hypercapnia. Other causes include disease of the spine, chest wall, muscles and nerves, obesity and sedation.
2. With a low Pco_2—this is seen with unilateral lung disease, such as pneumonia or collapse; with diffusion defects, such as oedema or fibrosis and with ventilation—perfusion inequality such as pulmonary embolism or asthma. It occurs because hyperventilation associated with malfunctioning of some alveolar-capillary units can lower the Pco_2 but cannot raise the arterial oxygen

saturation in blood coming from the normally functioning units because it is already 95% saturated.

Oxygen may be given freely. It will not affect hypoxia due to an intracardiac shunt. With diffusion defects Po_2 falls further with exertion. The Pco_2 may rise in the late stage of most of these conditions.

Effects of hypoxia
Haemoglobin is fully saturated at Po_2 levels above 10.5 kPa, but saturation falls off rapidly when Po_2 levels drop below 8 kPa. Certain factors reduce the saturation of haemoglobin at a given Po_2 (right shift of the Hb O_2 dissociation curve) and improve oxygen delivery to the tissues without greatly reducing oxygen uptake in the lungs. These include acidosis, hypercapnia and pyrexia. Rapid total correction of these conditions could therefore aggravate tissue hypoxia. Clinically, tachypnoea, tachycardia, restlessness, sweating, and finally cyanosis but not necessarily dyspnoea occur with hypoxia. Central cyanosis appears when the concentration of desaturated haemoglobin reaches 5 g per 100 ml. This normally occurs at a Po_2 of below 7 kPa, but will occur more easily if there is polycythaemia and is delayed if there is anaemia.

ALLERGY

Immunity is the process of protection of the body against foreign material. A foreign substance is one that is recognized by the body as 'not self'. It may come from outside, as with bacteria, or be intrinsic, as with an altered tissue component. Allergy or hypersensitivity is an increased immune response to foreign material, previously met. Tolerance is a less than normal response. The immune response is both humoral and cellular.

A complete antigen can stimulate lymphocytes to respond with a cellular reaction or to produce specific antibodies. It can specifically combine with these antibodies and provoke a tissue reaction. They are mainly larger size proteins. Incomplete antigens (haptens) are low molecular weight chemicals that do not evoke antibody production but can combine with specific antibody, though without resultant tissue reaction. A hapten conjugated with a carrier protein becomes a complete antigen. An allergen is an antigen involved in atopic allergy.

Antibodies are γ-globulins (p. 14) produced by lymphocytes. Lymphocytes are of two sorts, T cells which pass through the thymus and are concerned with cell-mediated immunity, and B cells which pass though gut-associated lymphoid tissue and produce antibodies. The lymphocytes produce IgM and differentiate to plasma cells which produce IgG (p. 15). Antigen–antibody complexes initiate tissue reaction through chemical mediators such as complement (p. 18) and histamine.

Types of Allergic Response
There are four main types of allergic response involved in different diseases. Any of the four types may be involved in drug reactions.

Type I (immediate hypersensitivity, anaphylactic) allergy
IgE antibody attaches to cell surfaces and sensitizes them to release histamine on combination with an external antigen. On prick testing with antigen, a weal appears and is maximal at fifteen minutes. A response to several antigens is found in the atopic state. Antihistamines but not corticosteroids cause false-negatives. This reaction is involved in anaphylaxis and atopic conditions.

Type II (cytotoxic) allergy
Circulating IgG or IgM antibody combines with cell membrane antigen and complement. This occurs in transfusion reactions and Goodpasture's syndrome. Skin testing is not appropriate.

Type III (Arthus, late immune complex) allergy
Circulating antigen–antibody immune complexes settle in lung and kidney and activate complement. Intradermal injection of allergen causes diffuse oedema and erythema, maximal at 6 hours. There may be a preceding Type I reaction. Positive results occur with bronchopulmonary aspergillosis and extrinsic allergic alveolitis such as bird fancier's lung. There may also be precipitins in the blood.

Type IV (delayed, cell-mediated) allergy
Antigens stimulate lymphocyte activity without antibody involvement. Intradermal injection of allergen causes induration, maximal at 48 hours. Tuberculin (p. 75), brucellin, lepromin and patch tests in contact dermatitis are of this nature. These tests have epidemiological and diagnostic use. They also use the ability of the lymphocyte

system to resist infection and all tests of this type may be negative with impaired lymphocyte function, e.g. Hodgkin's disease. Corticosteroid treatment suppresses this reaction.

Atopy

Atopic patients have a constitutional tendency to develop type I reactions to common allergens which provoke no response in normals. These allergens include pollens, moulds, feathers, animal danders, foods such as eggs, and mites in household dust. Atopic subjects have a high incidence of infantile eczema, hay fever, allergic rhinitis and asthma. Suggestive features are a family history, raised IgE levels, positive type I skin reactions to several allergens and eosinophilia in blood and respiratory tract secretion. Direct provocation tests to lung or nose are diagnostically useful but potentially dangerous.

CLINICAL PROBLEMS

Airways Obstruction

This occurs in asthma, emphysema and chronic bronchitis. In all three FEV_1, FVC, FEV_1/FVC and PEFR are low. Asthma is characterized by marked variability of the PEFR and FEV_1 over short periods, a 20% improvement with β-adrenergic stimulant drugs and evidence of atopy in some patients. In emphysema there is evidence of hyperinflation on X-ray, as with asthma, and the TLC is markedly raised. In wheezy chronic bronchitis there is often a history of smoking and productive cough. Variability is less than in asthma and the response to an inhaled anticholinergic drug (ipatropium) may be better than the response to a β-adrenergic stimulant.

Restrictive Disease

Typically FEV_1 and FVC are low but FEV_1/FVC is normal. This distinction from airways obstruction is blurred in severe disease of either sort. CXR can be normal, Po_2 may be low with a low Pco_2. TLC and TLCO are reduced. Progress is best monitored by changes in VC. Restrictive disease is seen with sarcoidosis, fibrosing alveolitis, allergic alveolitis and neoplastic infiltration.

Chronic Dyspnoea

If the cause of dyspnoea is uncertain after clinical examination and chest X-ray, the following conditions should be considered: asthma, emphysema, occult heart failure, diffuse pulmonary fibrosis and thromboembolic pulmonary hypertension (p. 173). An important step is to measure the pulse rate, ECG, PFT and blood gases before and after exertion. Simple observation during exertion may reveal asthma or psychogenic problems. Note that the PFT levels are abnormal in emphysema, even if the X-ray is not. Early diffuse pulmonary fibrosis may be difficult. Here the Po_2 falls with exertion and the TLCO and tests of lung compliance may be abnormal.

In combined cardiorespiratory pathology, the higher PEFR is above 250 l/min. and FEV_1 is above 1.5 l, the more likely is severe dyspnoea to be cardiac. As PEFR falls to 100 l/min. and FEV_1 to 1 l, the more likely is dyspnoea to be respiratory. An FVC below 50% of normal is likely to contribute to dyspnoea.

Pneumonia

In lobar pneumonia the chest X-ray shows a homogeneous opacity. Pulmonary infarction (p. 173) and infection secondary to obstruction such as neoplasm must be considered. The X-ray in bronchopneumonia shows patchy bilateral shadows and the condition occurs mostly in patients who are old, weak or have pre-existing lung disease. Gram-stained sputum smears (p. 201), sputum and blood culture, examination and culture of pleural fluid and serological tests are helpful in differential diagnosis.

Pneumococcal pneumonia is typically lobar, but bronchopneumonia can occur if there is debility or pre-existing lung disease. Staphylococcal pneumonia occurs with influenza and in diabetes. There is severe toxaemia and multiple abscesses can occur. *Klebsiella pneumoniae* usually invades the upper lobes and may cause abscess formation in patients with known lung disease. *Pseudomonas aeruginosa* causes a diffuse nodular bronchopneumonia of the lower lobes in patients with cystic fibrosis or on ventilators. Its presence in sputum does not prove a pathogenic role.

Anaerobic infection (p. 72) usually results from aspiration. Abscesses occur but cultures are often negative. Legionnaires' disease causes a severe pneumonia often with diarrhoea, confusion, abnormal liver function tests or hyponatraemia. Diagnosis is best made by an indirect serum immunofluorescent antibody test. Tuberculosis must always be considered. Here the sputum is often mucoid and there is no leucocytosis.

Pneumonia due to infection by mycoplasmae, rickettsiae or chlamydiae (p. 76) presents with an atypical picture. Systemic disturbance is more marked than respiratory features, though the chest X-ray may show a lobar or bronchopneumonic pattern. Sputum may be mucoid, with no leucocytosis in the blood. The diagnosis is confirmed by serological tests.

In debilitated and especially immunosuppressed patients, infection by cytomegalovirus (p. 84), or *Pneumocystis carinii*, and aspergillosis (p. 86) must be considered.

Chapter Twenty

DISEASES OF THE NERVOUS SYSTEM

BRAIN IMAGING

Skull X-ray
Erosion of the posterior clinoid is seen in raised intracranial pressure and also hypertension. Shift of a calcified pineal gland may indicate a space-occupying lesion. Bone destruction or cerebral calcification may be seen.

Echo-Encephalogram
Deviation of the midline structures can be detected when the pineal gland is not calcified.

Brain Scan
Uptake of injected isotope by the brain is measured by a gamma camera and analysed by computer. Rapid sequence photography after injection may show increased activity in a large vascular lesion or diminished perfusion with large vessel occlusion. Distribution of isotope 30 min. later is affected by changes in vascularity and the blood–brain barrier. Lesions at the base of the brain, in the posterior fossa or below 2 cm in diameter, are not well shown. The shape and site but not the nature of a lesion are determined. A negative scan is evidence against a space-occupying lesion, but false-positives and false-negatives can occur.
1. Tumour—a doubtful lesion becomes more positive with time.
2. Subdural haematoma—after two weeks, well shown as peripheral crescentic radioactivity.
3. Cerebral infarction—abnormality appears after a week and disappears in a few months.
4. Cerebral haemorrhage—abnormality lessens with time.

Computerized Tomography (CT)

This safe technique has, where available, largely replaced the brain scan and considerably reduced the need for invasive procedures such as air encephalography. It is indicated for all space-occupying lesions, e.g. neoplasms, abscesses and haemorrhages. It can differentiate between infarction and haemorrhage. Cerebral atrophy and hydrocephalus can be identified. It is very useful in severe head trauma. Posterior fossa lesions are less well shown. It is expensive and is not a routine screening procedure.

CEREBROSPINAL FLUID (CSF)

Lumbar puncture is essential when meningitis is suspected and is useful in subarachnoid haemorrhage, multiple sclerosis and Guillain-Barré syndrome. It is dangerous when space-occupying lesions are suspected, or when there is a bleeding tendency. It is not indicated in strokes.

Total Protein

Normal

Adults	0.15–0.40 g/l
Neonates	0.20–1.20 g/l
Elderly	0.15–0.50 g/l

Increase

Blood causes a rise of about 0.01 g/l for every 1000 red cells/mm^3.

1. 0.4–2.0 g/l—any pathology may cause this. Even a convulsion may raise the level to 0.80 g/l for a few weeks. In viral meningitis the protein level is usually below 1.0 g/l.
2. 2.0–5.0 g/l—this level is consistent with neoplasms, especially acoustic neuroma and also the conditions in 3.
3. Over 5.0 g/l—spinal obstruction, chronic meningitis and peripheral neuropathy.

The rise in protein often parallels the rise in white cells, but a disproportionate increase in protein occurs as follows:

1. Inflammatory disease—multiple sclerosis, syphilis.
2. Brain tumour.
3. Peripheral neuropathy—diabetes, Guillain-Barré syndrome.
4. Spinal block.

Globulin Levels

Analysis of CSF protein cannot be performed on bloody fluid. It is most useful in multiple sclerosis, but globulins are also abnormal in neurosyphilis, encephalitis, polyneuropathy, tumours and systemic lupus erythematosus. In these conditions electrophoresis can show an increase in IgG of restricted heterogeneity (oligoclonal). Gamma-globulin is normally less than 20% of total protein, and IgG is normally less than 14% of total protein (below 0.06 g/l).

Where electrophoresis is not available the Pándy test or the colloidal gold reaction may be useful. In the Pándy test, cloudiness with phenol suggests excess globulins provided that the total protein content is below 0.7 g/l. In the colloidal gold reaction (Lange curve) the reagent is precipitated by serial CSF dilutions and the amount of precipitation is graded 0–5. Raised γ-globulin concentrations increase precipitation in the less diluted tubes (paretic curve, early rise).

Glucose

0.5 ml is put into a fluoride tube.

Normal

Adults	2.7–4.4 mmol/l
Neonates	1.1–2.2 mmol/l
Infants and children	3.9–5.0 mmol/l

It is 0.5–1.0 mmol/l or 10–40% below the blood level which should always be measured simultaneously or an abnormality may be missed in a diabetic or a patient receiving i.v. glucose. Measurement is useful mainly in suspected meningitis. Normal levels are seen in most viral meningitides and cerebral abscess. Levels below 1.0 mmol/l usually occur in bacterial meningitis, rarely tuberculosis, but a normal CSF glucose does not completely exclude bacterial meningitis.

Moderate decrease (1.0–2.5 mmol/l)

1. Chronic meningitis, especially tuberculous or mycotic.
2. Any gross pleocytosis, such as with neoplasms or in sarcoidosis.
3. Viral meningitis, especially if there are many cells, e.g. in mumps and lymphocytic choriomeningitis.
4. Bacterial meningitis, especially if partly treated.

Cells

Normal

Adults	0– 5 white blood cells (WBC)/mm^3; 0– 10 red blood cells (RBC)/mm^3
Neonates	0–15 WBC/mm^3; 0–500 RBC/mm^3
Infants and children	0– 8 WBC/mm^3; 0– 10 RBC/mm^3

One WBC is added for every 500 RBC. Rarely a CSF is examined too early in a meningitis for many cells to appear or for the sugar to fall. Mononuclear cells usually predominate in viral and chronic disease and polymorphonuclear cells in acute bacterial disease, but exceptions do occur, so the cell type is not an absolute guide to the pathology. Cloudiness of the CSF does not appear until the WBC count exceeds 500/mm^3. Malignant cells must be sought in fresh specimens.

Red cells

Blood caused by a traumatic tap clears partly in the second specimen and there is no xanthochromia. After a subarachnoid haemorrhage xanthochromia appears in 4 hours and disappears in 2–4 weeks. Red cells appear within an hour and disappear in 3–7 days.

Polymorphonuclear cells

These predominate in infection due to pyogenic organisms. Counts may be low early, but over 10 000/mm^3 later. They may also predominate in:

1. Early viral meningitis, e.g. poliomyelitis.
2. Early tuberculosis.
3. Carcinomatous meningitis.

Mononuclear cells

Counts are usually below 200/mm^3.

1. Meningitis—viral (counts up to 1000/mm^3), tuberculous, leptospiral, fungal, and in association with sarcoidosis.
2. Encephalitis.
3. Demyelinating disease (usually below 30/mm^3).
4. Space-occupying lesion—abscess, tumour.
5. Syphilis.

Mixed pleocytosis
The extent of the pleocytosis and the predominant cell type varies. The following conditions should be considered:
1. Tuberculous meningitis (early).
2. Poliomyelitis (early).
3. Aseptic meningeal reaction—nearby sepsis or brain destruction. Seen in cerebral abscess, osteomyelitis of the skull and intracranial sinus thrombosis. CSF sugar is normal.
4. Subarachnoid haemorrhage—white cells appear later owing to meningeal irritation.

Serological Tests For Syphilis (p. 74)

Bacteriology
The film must be examined by an experienced person. Positive identification of organisms such as meningococci or tubercle bacilli may be made. A Gram stain may be positive when culture is negative because of previous antibiotics. Viral culture should be supplemented by culture of other secretions and serum antibodies.

ELECTROPHYSIOLOGY

Electroencephalography (EEG)
The EEG detects the electrical activity of the cerebral cortex and in general is used to investigate disturbed function such as epilepsy rather than structural abnormality.

The diagnosis of epilepsy is essentially clinical and the EEG is often quite normal between fits, whilst minor electrical abnormalities are seen in normal people. However, the spike-and-wave discharges of petit mal may be seen and the wave pattern may indicate whether epilepsy is secondary to a temporal lobe focus or a structural lesion elsewhere. Provocative procedures such as hyperventilation may be useful. The EEG can be useful in unexplained coma when fast rhythms suggestive of drug overdose or focal disturbance consistent with a structural lesion may be seen.

The EEG may be suggestive but not diagnostic of superficial tumours and vascular diseases.

Electronystagmography
Subclinical nystagmus, normally suppressed by ocular fixation, is

detected electrically using various stimuli, such as caloric tests. Lesions in the vestibular system and oculomotor lesions can be detected and brain stem pathology can be distinguished from peripheral lesions.

Audiometry
This is helpful to detect and distinguish between lesions of the middle ear, labyrinth and eighth cranial nerve. It is most helpful with Ménière's disease and cerebellopontine-angle tumours.

Evoked Potentials
Surface electrodes record the delay between a sensory stimulus and the resulting electric potentials in the central nervous system. Visual, followed by auditory and somatosensory tests are most used. Subclinical lesions in these pathways can be detected. Hysterical and unco-operative patients can be assessed. The tests are most used in suspected multiple sclerosis.

Electrodiagnosis of Nerve and Muscle Disease
The available techniques are used to distinguish between conditions affecting the muscles, the myoneural junction and the peripheral nerves. They can also locate the disease process more precisely.

Electromyography (EMG)
Muscles are sampled with a concentric needle electrode. In muscle disease the muscle is silent when the needle is inserted, and with contraction the number of motor units is normal but each potential is small and of short duration. Exceptions to this are myotonia, where the needle causes a prolonged run of potentials (dive-bomber pattern), and polymyositis, where nerve endings may be involved. In nerve disease there are spontaneous fibrillation potentials, and with muscle contraction the number of motor units is less owing to axon loss, but they may be larger due to sprouting of the remaining nerve fibres.

Nerve Conduction Velocity
The muscle action potential can be recorded when the motor nerve is stimulated or the action potential over the nerve can be recorded after sensory stimulation. The site of a peripheral nerve lesion, e.g. carpal tunnel, can be located when conduction velocity is delayed

due to demyelination. Proximal axon loss does not usually delay conduction.

Neuromuscular Transmission
Changes in the muscle action potential after repetitive motor nerve stimulation can distinguish between myasthenic syndromes.

CLINICAL PROBLEMS

Suspected Meningitis
The absence of pyrexia in the elderly does not preclude the diagnosis. A blood sugar and a blood culture are taken at the same time as the CSF. Cultures are also taken of any other possibly infected material. In the absence of a positive culture, diagnosis depends on the total clinical picture.

Aseptic Meningitis
Clinical meningitis with a polymorphonuclear or mixed pleocytosis, a low sugar and a negative culture is seen in:
1. Bacterial infection. Partly treated pyogenic and tuberculous meningitis are common causes. Unusual infections such as leptospirosis are considered.
2. Fungal infection—this is seen particularly with immunodeficiency. Indian-ink staining and appropriate culture are necessary.
3. Viral meningitis, e.g. poliomyelitis.
4. Parameningeal infection—brain abscess, ear infection.
5. Non-infective meningitis, e.g. carcinoma, sarcoidosis, chemical.
6. Bacterial endocarditis.

Tuberculous Meningitis (TBM)
This is usually a subacute progressive illness but may present more like an acute bacterial meningitis. When suspected, a careful search for tubercle bacilli is made on several CSF specimens. Culture results take some weeks and it may be advisable to start treatment in the absence of proof because the total clinical picture is suggestive. The typical CSF has a raised pressure, is clear or slightly cloudy and forms a clot on standing. The protein is raised (over 2 g/l), the sugar is low (1–2.3 mmol/l) and the cell count is 25–500/mm^3, mainly lymphocytes. Culture is negative. CWR is negative and there are no fungi. Evidence of tuberculosis elsewhere is sought by chest X-ray

and Mantoux test (p. 75). It is possible for the first CSF to be normal or contain mainly polymorphonuclear cells. In the absence of tubercle bacilli, the other causes of a mononuclear or mixed pleocytosis should be considered.

If available, computerized tomography and the demonstration of increased permeability of the blood–brain barrier by radioactive bromide or technetium is helpful. The relative concentrations of bromide in blood and CSF are in the ratio 3:1, and a ratio below 1.9:1 is consistent with TBM.

Multiple Sclerosis
The diagnosis is essentially clinical, but help may be obtained by study of CSF cells, proteins, serology, and by evoked potentials.

Subarachnoid Haemorrhage
Computerized tomography (CT) can demonstrate blood in the subarachnoid space. Where CT is unavailable or inconclusive, lumbar puncture is necessary, but this is contraindicated by hemiplegia, stupor or coma as coning may be precipitated. Irritation of the meninges may cause the WBC count to reach 500/mm^3 in a delayed lumbar puncture. If operation is possible, angiography should be performed.

Neuromuscular Disorders
The clinical diagnosis may be confirmed by techniques described above. Peripheral neuropathy is associated with widespread nerve conduction abnormalities. In motor neurone disease, EMG is useful. In polymyositis there are EMG and enzyme abnormalities (p. 123). In myotonia the EMG is abnormal. In muscular dystrophies the enzymes may be abnormal.

Muscle or nerve biopsy may be essential, but are best undertaken in a specialized unit.

Chapter Twenty One

KIDNEY DISEASES

The anatomy of the urinary tract is studied by radiological techniques and these may also indicate the pathology in conditions such as calculous disease, obstruction and pyelonephritis. Overall renal function is best measured by an assessment of the glomerular filtration rate (GFR). Isotope studies are the best guide to function in one kidney or part of a kidney. Specific tests are used for individual aspects of tubular function. Analysis of urine constituents indicates the presence of pathology and gives evidence about its nature. Abnormalities in the plasma also contribute to diagnosis.

URINARY TRACT IMAGING

The plain abdominal film is a preliminary to most other studies. It may indicate the size of the kidneys and the presence of calculi or nephrocalcinosis.

Intravenous Urogram (IVU)
This very useful technique gives information about the position, size and shape of the kidneys, the cortex and the pelvicalyceal system. The information it gives about the ureters and bladder is less reliable. In particular, bladder neoplasms are best detected by the cystoscope. Renal function is best assessed by isotope methods, as contrast density is affected by factors other than the GFR. Useful variations of the technique for special circumstances are possible and, in particular, high doses of contrast medium and tomography are important in renal failure. Multiple myeloma and diabetic nephropathy are relative contraindications to the IVU.

Other Radiological Techniques
Arteriography is used in the study of renal masses, hypertension, trauma, haematuria and loss of function of a kidney. Venography is

used for renal vein thrombosis and may be helpful in the study of a neoplasm. In micturating cystourethrography the bladder is filled with contrast medium through a catheter and films during micturition may demonstrate vesicoureteric reflux.

Urethrography is used for urethral lesions. Pyelography is an invasive technique less used now. It is done through a ureteric catheter (retrograde) or a needle inserted into the renal pelvis (antegrade) and is used in the study of ureteric lesions.

Computerized tomography can be used when i.v. urography and ultrasound have not satisfactorily demonstrated a renal mass, in obstructive uropathy and it also provides a non-invasive method of diagnosing renal vein thrombosis.

Ultrasonography
By this technique renal size can be measured, non-functioning kidneys are outlined, and cysts and hydronephrosis can be detected. It shows whether a tumour is cystic or solid, provided the cyst is not less than about 2 cm in diameter. It can detect the cysts of polycystic disease before urography. As it is not dependent on renal function, it is especially useful in renal failure.

Isotope Studies
Renography gives a curve of isotope activity against time. Activity over the kidneys depends on both rate of uptake and rate of excretion. Slow uptake occurs in renal artery stenosis and slow clearance in stasis or ureteric obstruction. Excretion delay due to stasis will clear with i.v. frusemide. The amount of residual urine in the bladder and vesicoureteric reflux can be measured. Orthoiodohippuric acid (Hippuran), which is excreted by both glomerular filtration and the tubules, is used for these techniques.

Diethylenetriamine-penta-acetic acid (DTPA) is useful for comparing the GFR in each kidney as it is excreted by glomerular filtration. Dimercaptosuccinic acid (DMSA) binds to the tubules and outlines the functioning areas of a kidney. An area which shows no function with DMSA may concentrate gallium if there is infection, infarction or tumour.

URINALYSIS
Screening for proteinuria is carried out by a dipstick test or less commonly by salicylsulphonic acid. However, tests on random

samples may give false-negatives with dilute urines and trace false-positive reactions with concentrated urines. Simultaneous measurement of the random urine creatinine concentration corrects for this and the protein concentration expressed as mg protein per 10 mmol creatinine approximates to the total daily urine protein excretion. Alternatively, daily protein excretion may be measured by a full 24-hour collection.

Dipsticks

These (e.g. Albustix) are impregnated with an acid–base indicator which changes colour in the presence of protein. They detect protein in concentrations down to 40 mg/l. They are more sensitive to albumin than globulin or haemoglobin and will miss Bence Jones protein and tubular proteins. False positives occur with alkaline urines including those contaminated by detergents.

Salicylsuphonic acid

Five drops of a 25% solution is added to 5 ml of urine and the result graded from 0 – 4+. Bence Jones protein and globulins are more likely to be detected than with Albustix. Trace positive reactions are seen at protein concentrations of down to 50 mg/l. False-positive results are seen when the urine contains X-ray media, excessive urates, PAS, tolbutamide or considerable penicillin.

Significance of Proteinuria

The proteins found in the urine in glomerular disease are albumin and larger proteins. In tubular disease smaller proteins are lost. When haemoglobin, myoglobin or immunoglobulin light chains appear in the circulation an overflow proteinuria occurs.

Normal

Adults	< 150 mg per 24 h.
	Daytime excretion does not exceed 100 mg/l.
Children	< 100 mg per 24 h.

Persistent proteinuria, not purely postural, implies urinary tract disease, in the absence of hypertension and cardiac failure. If proteinuria remains over 500 mg per 24 h after these have been controlled, additional renal pathology is likely.

Functional (reversible) proteinuria
Excretion is less than 500 mg per 24 h, mainly albumin, and stops with recovery. It occurs in acute illness in the absence of renal disease, especially heart failure and fever and also after severe exertion.

Postural proteinuria
The urine passed in recumbency is protein free (below 20 mg/l). On the night before the test it is best to pass and discard the urine after the first two hours of recumbency, collecting the first urine in the morning. Proteinuria should only be accepted as purely postural if the early morning urine is protein free on two occasions, daily excretion is below 1.2 g during normal activity and the urine depósit and serum creatinine are normal. This condition occurs in 3% of normal adolescents. It should be noted that all proteinuria is lessened by recumbency and serious nephropathy may rarely present with initially purely postural proteinuria.

Renal disease without proteinuria
Proteinuria is often absent in diseases which do not primarily involve the glomeruli. Benign nephrosclerosis is a common cause of mild renal impairment without proteinuria in older people. Other causes include surgical and congenital disease and interstitial nephritis. Even in glomerular disease proteinuria may be intermittently absent.

Heavy proteinuria
Glomerular damage is likely to be present if proteinuria exceeds 1 g per 24 h. Excretion rates over 3.5 g per 24 h (0.05 g/kg per 24 h) are consistent with the nephrotic syndrome.

Urine Electrophoresis
With glomerular disease there is mainly albumin and γ-globulin. If proteinuria is non-selective, macroglobulin and β-lipoproteins appear also. With tubular disease proteinuria is not heavy and α_2-globulin occurs commonly. Bence Jones protein appears as a sharp peak near the γ-globulin region. Haemoglobin (p. 258) and myoglobin are usually detected by spectroscopy but may be noted by urine electrophoresis.

Protein Selectivity

The clearance (C) of a large molecule, e.g. IgG, is compared with that of a small molecule, e.g. transferrin (T).

$$\text{Selectivity} = \frac{C_{IgG}}{C_T} .$$

As we are comparing clearances, the volume term cancels out, and the test can be done on a random aliquot of urine.

$$\text{Selectivity} = \frac{U_{IgG} \times P_T}{P_{IgG} \times U_T}$$

where U = urine concentration; P = plasma concentration.

A ratio of < 0.15 is highly selective and suggests that the glomerular membrane is impermeable to high molecular weight proteins. A ratio of above 0.30 is poorly selective, indicating leakage of a wide range of proteins. The main use of the test is in the childhood nephrotic syndrome, where a high selectivity suggests a steroid responsive condition.

Blood

Dipstick tests are based on the peroxidase-like activity of haemoglobin. They are more sensitive to lysed than intact red cells. False-positives occur with infected urine and when there is myoglobinuria. Positive results should be checked by microscopy, but lysed red cells in hypotonic urine can be missed by this method when the dipstick is positive. False-negatives occur in concentrated urines because red cells do not lyse and they also occur if there is a high concentration of ascorbic acid.

Centrifuged Deposit

Normal

Red cells 0–1 per high-power field (hpf, $\times$ 40); white cells 0–2 per hpf, 0–5 per hpf in the uncatheterized female. Hyaline casts are occasionally seen. An excess of red cells indicates bleeding somewhere in the urinary tract. They are likely to have a glomerular origin if there is heavy proteinuria, the IVU is normal and a skilled observer can see marked variation of size and haemoglobin content with a phase-contrast microscope.

White cells (WBC) are recognized by their granular cytoplasm and lobed nuclei. They occur with inflammation, vascular disease and any acute illness.

Tubular cells are larger than WBC and have oval nuclei. They occur in acute renal failure, toxic nephropathy and with analgesics. Large numbers of squamous epithelial cells indicate vulval contamination and invalidate cell counts. A completely normal count in a concentrated morning urine is a good piece of evidence against renal disease. Slightly abnormal counts must be interpreted with caution. Malignant cells are more likely to be discovered in carcinoma of the bladder and ureter than of the kidney.

Casts

These are formed of coagulated protein, with or without cellular elements, and usually imply increased cell or protein excretion. Hyaline casts are featureless and not necessarily pathological as they can occur with exertion, fever and diuretics. Granular casts can appear with any acute illness but frequently imply some kind of renal pathology. Red cell casts occur in acute glomerulonephritis, malignant hypertension and polyarteritis nodosa. White cell casts are characteristic of pyelonephritis, but occur with any interstitial nephritis and even with glomerulonephritis.

Bacteriology

Screening tests for urinary infection are not very reliable. A stick test which utilizes nitrate reduction and an azo-dye is available. If more than one organism per high-power field is seen in Gram-stained, unspun, fresh urine, bacteriuria may be suspected, but vaginal contamination gives false-positives and coccal infections are missed.

The standard test is the midstream urine specimen (MSU), obtained after retracting the prepuce or labia and washing the glans or vulva with sterile water. It is reliable in the circumcised male, less so in the female. False-positives are seen when the specimen is not refrigerated or sent to the laboratory without delay. This problem may be avoided by immediate culture on a dipslide. False-negatives occur if antiseptic gets into the specimen jar or the patient has recently been given an antibiotic. Infection is more likely to be present if a single organism is grown. In doubtful cases quantitative counts are helpful. These can be obtained even in general practice by dipping a prepared slide into the urine and sending it to the laboratory. Each organism develops into a colony which can be counted by eye.

E. coli and *Staph. saprophyticus* are common causes of urinary infection in general practice. *Staph. aureus, Strep. pyogenes* Group B and enterococci also cause infection, but growth in culture may be scanty. In hospitals mixed infections with resistant organisms, e.g. *Pr. mirabilis, Kl. aerogenes* and *Ps. pyocyanea*, are found. Diphtheroids, α-haemolytic streptococci and lactobacilli are not urinary pathogens. It may be difficult to decide whether an organism giving a scanty growth on culture is a pathogen or a contaminant. A suprapubic aspiration will confirm whether the organism is present in the bladder.

Patients with dysuria and pyuria usually have infective urethritis or cystitis even if the culture is sterile. Infection with *Chlamydia*, gonorrhoea, candida, trichomonas and tuberculosis must be sought by appropriate methods. Patients with dysuria, a normal urine deposit and negative culture may have candida infection, traumatic urethritis or vaginitis. Involvement of the upper urinary tract is suggested by pyrexia, loin pain, an abnormal urogram, white cell casts in the urine or recurrence of infection with the same organism within 14 days of treatment.

Asymptomatic bacteriuria is defined as a heavy growth (over 10^5/ml) of a single organism in the absence of pus cells and symptoms. It is important in pregnancy, as pyelonephritis may follow.

GLOMERULAR FILTRATION RATE (GFR)

This is assessed by clearance studies and by the plasma creatinine and urea concentrations. It correlates well with the overall ability of the kidney to maintain the 'milieu intérieur'.

Clearances

The clearance of a substance (C_S) is the volume of plasma (ml) from which that substance is totally removed or cleared by the kidney or other organ in one minute.

$$C_S \text{ (ml/min.)} = \text{Excretion/min.} \div \text{Plasma conc./ml} = \frac{U_S \times V}{P_S}$$

where U_S = urinary concentrations of S (per ml)
$\quad\quad P_S$ = plasma concentrations of S (per ml)
$\quad\quad V$ = urine volume (per min.)

Most substances are only partly cleared from the plasma by the kidney, so their clearance values are notional. Where a substance is freely permeable through the glomerular capillaries and neither reabsorbed nor secreted by the tubules its clearance is equal to the GFR. This applies to inulin, vitamin B12 and, with some qualification, to creatinine. A problem with all these methods is the need for accurate, timed urine collection.

Isotope GFR Estimations

One method of estimating the GFR without the need for urine collection is to calculate it from the disappearance rate of a radioactive isotope of a substance such as vitamin B12 or chromium edetate from the blood. Chemical estimations are also bypassed and the GFR is calculated by exponential analysis of the disappearance rate of the isotope from the plasma.

Creatinine Clearance (Ccr)

Normal

Adult males	91–119 ml/min./1.73 m^2
Adult females	77–113 ml/min./1.73 m^2
Neonates	40– 65 ml/min./1.73 m^2
Children	adult levels (per 1.73 m^2) by 2 yr
Elderly	After 40 yr, decreases by 6 ml/min. per decade.
Pregnancy	Increase by 50%

It is estimated on a 24 hour urine collection using the equation:

$$Ccr\ (ml/min.) = \frac{Ucr\ (\mu mol/l) \times V\ (ml)}{Pcr\ (\mu mol/l) \times 1440}$$

Note that there are 1440 minutes in 24 hours and that urine and plasma creatinine levels must both be expressed in μmol. The 24-hour collection is best as it reduces errors related to bladder emptying, but it remains liable to problems or incomplete collection. It is sufficient to take one serum creatinine measurement during the day.

Ccr gives a good estimation of the GFR, with some reservations. It is higher than the GFR as measured by the insulin clearance, the reference method, because of some tubular secretion, which occurs especially with nephrotic syndrome, renal failure and corticosteroid treatment. It may be reduced by drugs that affect the tubular handling of creatinine, e.g. cimetidine, high-dose salicylate, cephalosporins and trimethoprim.

Urea Clearance

The urea clearance is about 50% lower than the creatinine clearance because of urea reabsorption in the distal nephron. Generally this test is not useful, but in advanced renal failure there is an osmotic diuresis in the remaining nephrons and in these circumstances the urea clearance approximates to the creatinine clearance and both should be measured on the same blood and 24-hour urine specimen to assess the GFR. It is calculated as for creatinine, but we are dealing in mmol not μmol.

Urine Creatinine

This is sometimes measured as an approximate test of the completeness of a urine collection. It is also possible to express excretion of enzymes, proteins, or hormones in terms of units per mmol creatinine rather than units per 24 h.

Normal

Adult males	7 – 18 mmol per 24 h
Adult females	5.3 – 16 mmol per 24 h
Children	71 –195 μmol/kg per 24 h

Serum Creatinine (Scr)

Normal
Clotted blood, preferably taken fasting in the morning, as levels are 10% higher later.

Adult males	65–115 μmol/l
Adult females	55–100 μmol/l
Infants	20– 65 μmol/l
Children	30– 80 μmol/l
Elderly	see below.

Most automated methods overestimate the plasma creatinine by about 0.14 because of other chromogens.

The serum level is inversely proportional to the clearance, as is seen from the expression:

$$\text{Clearance} = \text{urinary output} \div \text{serum concentration}$$

As urinary output is constant in stable conditions, a doubling of the serum creatinine implies a halving of the creatinine clearance, so that it is the standard method of monitoring GFR in renal failure once the clearance has been determined. However, creatinine production is proportional to muscle mass, so serum levels are lower in women, the elderly, the wasted and the small. Therefore, isolated values are not reliable. Tiny old ladies may have apparently normal serum creatinine levels despite marked renal impairment. Scr is also not a sensitive guide to the onset of impairment of renal function, as a fall in the creatinine clearance to 50% will cause a doubling of the serum creatinine, but the latter may still remain within the wide range of normal. It is a better guide than plasma urea to the GFR because it is less affected by extrarenal factors, though it does rise slightly with increased protein intake.

It is possible to calculate the creatinine clearance per 1.73 m^2 from the serum creatinine concentration. The formulae are more reliable in children than adults. They are not reliable when there is wasting or obesity.

Adult males
$$\frac{1.23(140 - \text{age}) \times \text{Wt (kg)}}{\text{Serum creatinine } (\mu\text{mol/l})}$$

Adult females
$$\frac{1.04\,(140 - \text{age}) \times \text{Wt (kg)}}{\text{Serum creatinine } (\mu\text{mol/l})}$$

Children
$$\frac{\text{Height (cm)} \times 62}{\text{Serum creatinine } (\mu\text{mol/l})}$$

Serum Urea

Normal

Adult males	2.1–7.0 mmol/l
Adult females	1.8–6.6 mmol/l
Children	1.8–5.5 mmol/l

| Elderly | 3.1–9.5 mmol/l |
| Pregnancy | a fall by up to a third. |

The serum urea depends partly on the urea clearance, which is related to the GFR, and partly on the rate of urea production from the catabolism of ingested protein and body tissue. It is therefore a good measure of the overall balance between the load placed on the kidneys and the ability of the kidneys to deal with it, but it is not a good measure of renal function as such because it is affected by so many factors. Also, it is a poor measure of minor degrees of renal impairment because it can double in an individual and still remain within normal limits because the range for the population is so wide.

Increase (azotaemia)
1. Reduced excretion—usually owing to a reduced glomerular filtration rate, whether from renal, pre-renal or post-renal failure, but also due to increased reabsorption in water depletion.
2. Catabolism of absorbed protein—high protein diet, gastrointestinal haemorrhage.
3. Catabolism of endogenous protein—fever, infection, trauma, haemorrhage.
4. Drugs—tetracyclines and corticosteroids increase catabolism; diuretics and β-adrenergic blocking drugs can cause pre-renal failure; many drugs can cause renal damage.

Decrease
1. Anabolic states—infancy and pregnancy. Apparently normal levels may be pathological. In pregnancy it is usually < 4.5 mmol/l.
2. Low protein diet—alcoholism.
3. Liver failure—reduced synthesis.
4. I.v. infusions—ECF expansion raises the GFR and reduces tubular reabsorption of urea. In these circumstances the blood urea may not reflect the severity of renal impairment.

Serum Urea:Creatinine Ratio
The serum urea (in μmol/l) is normally 50–100 times the serum creatinine concentration (also in μmol/l). Changes in this ratio have some diagnostic significance.

Increase
1. Protein catabolism.
2. Sodium and water depletion—e.g. diuretics.
3. Cardiac failure.

Decrease
1. Reduced urea concentration (p. 231).
2. Raised creatinine concentration—dialysis, drugs blocking creatinine secretion (p. 229), rhabdomyolysis.

TUBULAR FUNCTION

Proximal Tubular Function
The proximal tubule reabsorbs filtered glucose, amino acids, sodium bicarbonate, phosphate, uric acid and potassium. In Fanconi's syndrome variable proximal tubular defects are seen, as well as distal tubular defects on occasions. There is, in particular, a heavy non-specific amino aciduria, glycosuria and phosphaturia. Hypokalaemia, hypouricaemia, acidosis and tubular proteinuria also occur. The blood urea rises only if there is fluid depletion or the disease progresses to destroy nephrons.

Causes of Fanconi's syndrome

Congenital. It may be the presenting feature of cystinosis, Lowe's syndrome and medullary cystic disease, as well as idiopathic Fanconi's syndrome. It also occurs in Wilson's disease (p. 135), galactosaemia and glycogen storage disease.

Acquired. Myelomatosis, amyloidosis, heavy proteinuria, Sjögren's syndrome and other autoimmune conditions, poisoning by heavy metals (lead, mercury, cadmium), phenols, or outdated tetracycline.

Glucose
A glucose tolerance test is necessary to distinguish renal glycosuria from impaired glucose tolerance. Renal glycosuria may be an isolated congenital abnormality or part of a proximal tubular syndrome. In pregnancy it is related to the rise in GFR.

Amino Acids
The various causes of aminoaciduria are grouped as follows:
1. Non-specific aminoaciduria — Fanconi's syndrome.
2. Specific tubular defects, e.g. cystinuria — there is a leak only of the dibasic amino acids, cystine, lysine, arginine and ornithine. Cystine can be detected by a nitroprusside test and cystinuria causes radio-opaque renal and bladder stones.
3. Overflow aminoaciduria — tubular reabsorption is normal but plasma levels are high because of a metabolic defect, e.g. phenylketonuria.

Phosphate
Renal phosphaturia may be suspected when phosphate is present in the urine despite a low serum level and in the absence of a non-renal cause (p. 54).
1. Renal tubular defects — Fanconi's syndrome, hereditary hypophosphataemic rickets, renal tubular acidosis.
2. Primary hyperparathyroidism.
3. Secondary hyperparathyroidism — usually due to vitamin D deficiency.

The Distal Nephron
The nephron beyond the proximal tubule is involved in urine acidification, sodium reabsorption and urine concentration. Damage causes hyperchloraemic acidosis, sodium depletion and polyuria. It is seen with obstructive uropathy, interstitial nephritis and several of the diseases which primarily affect the proximal tubule.

Urine Osmolality and Specific Gravity
Isotonic urine has a specific gravity of 1.010 and an osmolality of 300 mosmol/kg. Maximum urinary osmolality is about 1300 mosmol/kg (specific gravity 1.038). Very approximately a change in a specific gravity of 0.003 equals a change in osmolality of 100 mosmol/kg.

Specific gravity is a less accurate measure of concentrating power than osmolality because the latter depends only on the number of solute particles, whereas specific gravity is affected by their weight as well. Thus relatively large molecules which are still small enough to pass through the glomerulus will raise the specific gravity considerably but affect the osmolality much less. These include glucose, some proteins, X-ray media, mannitol and some low molecular weight dextrans. A false low value is seen when the urine is measured above room temperature. A random early morning urine specific gravity of 1020 (700 mosmol/kg) or more in the absence of sugar or protein excludes a serious concentrating defect. In the presence of oliguria, a hypertonic urine suggests ECF depletion.

Urine Concentration Test

Solid food and no liquid is allowed from 6.00 p.m. and three urines are measured for osmolality and specific gravity at 9.00, 10.00 and 11.00 a.m. the following morning. The test is stopped as soon as the osmolality reaches 800 mosmol/kg (sp. gr. 1024), which is normal, or earlier if the patient loses 5% of body weight.

Normal result
Urine osmolality > 800 mosmol/kg
Plasma osmolality < 300 mosmol/kg
Urine flow < 0.5 ml/min.
Urine:plasma osmolality ratio > 2.0.

Abnormal result
1. Diabetes insipidus (DI) — all four criteria are abnormal. Vasopressin (Pitressin) corrects pituitary, not nephrogenic, DI. If the patient is given intranasal synthetic vasopressin and allowed to drink at 11.00 a.m., the urine will concentrate in pituitary DI.
2. Psychogenic polydipsia — the result is normal. If there is illicit drinking, the urine does not concentrate, but the plasma osmolaltiy does not rise.
3. Distal tubular defects — hypokalaemia, hypercalcaemia, interstitial nephritis, obstructive uropathy, nephrogenic diabetes inspidus.
4. Miscellaneous — reduced concentration is seen in salt depletion owing to a lack of antidiuretic hormone, in diabetes mellitus and advanced renal failure due to osmotic diuresis and, in protein depletion due to reduced medullary tonicity, also in sicklaemia and with lithium or demeclocycline.

The main use of the test is in the diagnosis of diabetes insipidus due to posterior pituitary disease. It is also useful to demonstrate that polyuria is due to psychogenic polydipsia. Polyuria as a presenting complaint is usually seen only with diabetes mellitus, nephrogenic and pituitary diabetes insipidus.

Acidification

Acidosis of renal origin is usually due to renal failure, sometimes due to inability to lower the urinary pH in the distal tubule and rarely due to inability to reabsorb bicarbonate in the proximal tubule. With distal tubular defects there is always an abnormal response to ammonium chloride, but with proximal defects it may be normal. In tubular defects there is a hyperchloraemic acidosis and the main causes are:

1. Distal tubular diseases (p. 237).
2. Proximal tubular disease — some have also a distal effect.
3. Primary renal tubular acidosis — it occurs in children and adults and is associated with rickets, nephrocalcinosis, calculi and electrolyte depletion. Most cases are due to a distal renal tubular defect.

Acidification test

Ammonium chloride 0.1 g/kg in gelatine capsules is taken and the urine is collected under liquid paraffin in hourly aliquots for six hours, transferring the urine to the laboratory for testing as quickly as possible.

The pH should fall below 5.3 within three hours. The test is unnecessary if the pH of a random fresh urine sample is below 5.3. If the plasma bicarbonate does not fall by 4 mmol/l, the ammonium chloride has not been absorbed. The test is contraindicated by liver disease and if the urine is alkaline despite a systemic acidosis.

Sodium

Polyuria and continued urinary sodium loss (over 30 mmol/l) in a fluid-depleted patient suggests tubular dysfunction, severe renal disease or adrenal failure (p. 29).

PERCUTANEOUS RENAL BIOPSY

This is only carried out in specialized units where the information obtainable can be correctly interpreted. It is contraindicated by bleeding disorders, uncontrolled hypertension, an unco-operative patient, or a single kidney. The indications are:

1. Proteinuria in excess of 1 g per 24 h or associated with an abnormal centrifuged deposit, especially microscopic haematuria or if the GFR is also reduced.

2. Systemic disease with renal involvement, e.g. vasculitis, amyloidosis, connective tissue disease.
3. Acute renal failure, if unexplained.

CLINICAL PROBLEMS

Causes of Renal Disease
Some of the numerous causes of renal pathology may be loosely grouped as follows. Note that hypertension and infection may cause or may follow renal damage.
1. Glomerular disease.
2. Interstitial nephritis.
3. Vascular disease.
4. Surgical disease.

Investigation of Renal Disease
Renal disease is usually suspected when proteinuria, an abnormal deposit, urinary infection, azotaemia, hypertension or calculi are discovered. The basic investigation will include measurement of urine protein excretion, examination of the centrifuged deposit, urine culture, and measurement of serum creatinine and electrolytes, followed by i.v. urography (IVU). A raised serum creatinine means that both kidneys are damaged. Hypercalcaemia is usually a cause of renal failure rather than the consequence of it (p. 58). Hyperuricaemia unless very severe is a consequence, not a cause, of renal failure. Added to a careful history and examination, the above investigations are likely to indicate the type of pathology present.

Glomerular disease
This includes the various types of idiopathic glomerulonephritis, e.g. membranous, proliferative and sclerotic conditions and glomerulonephritis secondary to systemic disease, such as vasculitis and SLE. Diabetes mellitus and amyloidosis commonly involve the kidneys.

Proteinuria may be heavy. The IVU is usually normal. Red cell casts occur in acute glomerulonephritis, vasculitis and malignant hypertension. Further investigations may include serum and urine protein electrophoresis, serum complement, immunoglobulin and antinuclear factor estimation. Renal biopsy may be diagnostic.

Interstitial nephritis

Interstitial nephritides include bacterial pyelonephritis, calculous disease, hypercalcaemia, analgaesic nephropathy, obstructive uropathy, polycystic disease, and allergic drug reactions.

Evidence of tubular dysfunction predominates. There may be hyperchloraemic acidosis, excessive sodium loss and a concentration defect causing nocturia. Hypertension and loss of renal function also occur. There is more likely to be a difference in the function of each kidney than with glomerular disease. Pyuria is usual and the IVU may be abnormal.

Protein loss is due to a failure of tubular reabsorption, not glomerular leak. It is less than 1 g per 24 h. Albustix may be negative when salicylsulphonic acid is positive, as globulins appear in the urine including β2-microglobulin.

A careful history will suggest drug-induced disease. Allergic manifestations such as fever, rash, eosinophilia and eosinophils in the urine are often present, but may be absent, especially following the use of non-steroidal anti-inflammatory drugs. Renal biopsy is diagnostic.

Vascular disease

The vascular diseases include benign and malignant hypertension, and vascular occlusion. If renal damage is secondary to essential hypertension, the IVU is likely to be normal and proteinuria disappears with control of hypertension. Renal artery stenosis may be suspected when one kidney is small, but it must be diagnosed by angiography.

Surgical disease

Conditions remediable by surgery, e.g. obstruction, stones and neoplasms, are diagnosed initially by urography.

Severe Renal Failure

There are three main decisions to be made. Is the renal failure acute or chronic? Is it due to intrinsic renal disease or fluid depletion (pre-renal), or obstruction (post-renal)? These factors may be combined. If there is intrinsic renal disease what is its nature? It is especially important to exclude pre-renal and post-renal factors because of their remediable nature.

Acute or chronic renal failure

Chronic renal failure may be suggested by the history or previous records, which may not be immediately available, small kidneys demonstrated by imaging techniques, normochromic anaemia, evidence of azotaemic osteodystrophy (p. 56) or evidence of long-standing hypertension. Acute exacerbation of chronic renal failure by fluid depletion is common.

Obstructive uropathy

In the absence of a full bladder, ureteric obstruction by neoplasm or stones must still be considered. A high urine output does not exclude it. Ultrasound and urography will usually demonstrate obstruction, but retrograde pyelography may be necessary. Digital rectal and vaginal examination must be performed. The urine deposit is often normal.

Fluid depletion

Renal failure due to fluid depletion is readily reversible before acute tubular necrosis supervenes. There will be signs of ECF depletion (p. 30). Urine sodium is < 20 mmol/l. Urine osmolality is > 500 mosmol/kg and urine specific gravity is high. The urine to serum urea ratio is > 8. Urine microscopy is usually normal. Urine flow increases with fluid replacement, mannitol 20 g and frusemide 250 mg i.v.

Acute tubular necrosis (ATN)

This is the most common cause of acute renal failure in adults, but not children. There is usually a history of infection, shock or exposure to drugs or toxic agents. Milder cases may not be oliguric.

The following features help to differentiate ATN from oliguria due to ECF depletion. Urine microscopy reveals protein and casts. Urine osmolality is < 350 mosmol/kg. Urine sodium is > 60 mmol/l. The urine to serum urea ratio is < 4. There is no response to volume expansion, mannitol or frusemide 250 mg i.v. If frusemide has been given, urine sodium concentration is not a useful guide and the other urinary findings are also less useful if there is pre-existing renal disease.

Renal biopsy is indicated only if there is doubt about the renal pathology.

Acute interstitial nephritis

This is often due to non-steroidal anti-inflammatory drugs, but occurs with antibiotics and other drugs.

Acute glomerulonephritis

Haematuria, red blood cell casts and heavy proteinuria are likely. Hypertension and oedema are common.

Evidence of streptococcal infection, serum complement abnormalities (p. 18) and antiglomerular basement membrane antibodies may be present. There may also be evidence of systemic vasculitis or autoimmune disease.

Calculous Disease

Stones are diagnosed by i.v. urography. Uric acid calculi may be radiolucent. Recurrent stone formation may be associated with the following abnormalities: a high serum urate or calcium; increased urinary calcium, uric acid or oxalate excretion; impaired urine acidification, detected by monitoring urine pH or an acidification test; urinary tract abnormality associated with persistent infection. Chemical analysis of the stone is helpful.

Chapter Twenty Two

DISEASES OF THE RED BLOOD CELLS

ANAEMIA

Anaemia is usually recognized by a fall in the haemoglobin concentration, but this may not be seen in acute blood loss or ECF depletion and the hydraemia of pregnancy lowers the haemoglobin without always causing anaemia. The red cell volume is about 2000 ml in an adult and the red cell lifespan is about 120 days. This means that 16–20 ml of red cells are destroyed and the same quantity of cells are replaced each day. Either reduced red cell production or increased loss causes anaemia. In the latter case the resulting tissue hypoxia stimulates increased red cell production in the bone marrow by inducing the release of erythropoietin from the kidney.

Classification of Anaemia
The numerous causes may be classified according to cell size (p. 243) or aetiology. Often an anaemia has more than one cause.
1. Increased red cell loss — haemolysis, bleeding.
2. Reduced red cell production — nutritional deficiencies, marrow infiltration, drug induced, systemic disease.

Investigation of Anaemia
The haemoglobin concentration and the red cell indices measured by an automatic blood counter usually provide the initial diagnosis and assessment of anaemia. Red cell indices indicate only the average characteristics of the whole cell population and can miss qualitative changes and changes affecting a minority of cells. A careful assessment of the formed elements in the peripheral blood film is therefore the next step.

Small hypochromic cells suggest iron deficiency in Caucasians, but may be due to a haemoglobinopathy in other groups. A macrocytosis suggests megaloblastic anaemia, but has other causes (p. 243). Polychromasia suggests a reticulocytosis which may be due to haemolysis or blood loss. Bone marrow failure should be considered in a normocytic, normochromic anaemia not associated with acute blood loss.

Bone marrow examination must be considered in any anaemia where the cause is not readily apparent and particularly if there is neutropenia, thrombocytopenia or a leucoerythroblastic picture.

RED BLOOD CELL INDICES

Electronic counters are used to count red cells and measure their size accurately. Whole blood in a sequestrene tube is used.

Haemoglobin (Hb)

Normal

Adult males	13–18 g/dl
Adult females	12.0–17 g/dl
Neonates	17–20 g/dl
Infants (3 months)	10.5–12.0 g/dl
(1 year)	11.0–12.5 g/dl
Children (5 years)	12–13 g/dl
(> 10 years)	as for adults
Elderly females	11.5–16.0 g/dl
Pregnancy	lowest at 32 weeks, but not below 10.5 g/dl

The blood film or the red cell indices may indicate mild anaemia even when the Hb is still within the normal range.

Packed Cell Volume (PCV, Haematocrit)

Normal
Calculated from the cell count multiplied by the mean cell volume measured by electronic displacement.

Adult males	0.41–0.53 (41–53%)
Adult females	0.36–0.46
Neonates	0.45–0.67 (capillary sample)
Infants	0.28–0.42
Children	0.35–0.45

Direct measurement of the PCV by centrifugation is more precise but overestimates slightly because of trapped plasma, especially in iron deficiency. It is useful in the assessment of polycythaemia.

Red Cell Count (RCC)

Normal

Adult males	$4.5–6.5 \times 10^{12}/l$
Adult females	$3.9–5.6 \times 10^{12}/l$
Neonates (full term, cord blood)	$4.0–6.0 \times 10^{12}/l$
Infants (3 months)	$3.2–4.8 \times 10^{12}/l$
(1 year)	$3.6–5.2 \times 10^{12}/l$
Children	$4.0–5.4 \times 10^{12}/l$

Only electronic counting is accurate enough to be useful.

Mean Cell Volume (MCV)

Normal

Adults	84–99 fl (μm^3)
Neonates	95–121 fl
Infants	70–86 fl
Children	77–95 fl
Pregnancy	a rise of 4 fl after first trimester

Only electronic methods are useful. A low MCV indicates microcytosis, often an early sign of iron deficiency. A high MCV indicates macrocytosis. Anisocytosis or changes affecting a minority of cells will not be detected.

Mean Cell Haemoglobin (MCH)

Normal

Adults	26–35 pg
Neonates	28–42 pg
Infants	a gradual fall from birth to 24–30 pg at 1 year
Children	23–34 pg

The MCH is derived from Hb ÷ RCC and is accurate when electronic counters are used. A fall in the MCH is then a sensitive index of hypochromia or microcytosis. It can therefore be a useful non-specific test for iron deficiency. A rise in the MCH is seen in macrocytosis.

Mean Cell Haemoglobin Concentration (MCHC)

Normal
Electronic counter   32–36 g/dl
Manual measurement   30–36 g/dl

MCHC is derived from Hb ÷ PCV and is a good sign of hypochromia where the PCV is measured directly, but it is less useful with electronic counters, with which it falls only in severe hypochromia and overhydration and rises in severe dehydration.

Carboxyhaemoglobin
Normal   below 1%
Smokers   up to 8%

Symptoms may appear at a concentration of 10%.

THE PERIPHERAL BLOOD FILM

Changes in Size and Shape

Microcytosis
Small cells of normal or less thickness, often also hypochromic. Mainly seen in chronic iron deficiency and thalassaemia, and also in chronic systemic disease when they are usually normochromic.

Macrocytosis
Large cells. Seen in megaloblastic anaemia, even before Hb falls, reticulocytosis (p. 245), liver disease, hypothyroidism, aplastic anaemia, alcoholism, and with azathioprine and cyclophosphamide. A high haemoglobin with a macrocytosis is suggestive of alcohol abuse.

Anisocytosis
Abnormal variation in size. A non-specific change, sometimes marked in megaloblastic anaemia.

Spherocytosis
Small cells of increased thickness. Hereditary spherocytosis and other haemolytic diseases.

Poikilocytosis
Variation in shape. Several disorders associated with abnormal erythropoiesis or haemolysis.

Elliptocytosis
Oval cells. Seen in iron deficiency, hereditary elliptocytosis and, rarely, any severe anaemia.

Crenation
Contracted cells with regular projections. Usually an artefact due to drying. Sometimes seen in dysproteinaemia.

Acanthocytes
Irregular cells with helmet or triangular shape and burr cells with spiny projections. They occur in haemolysis due to drugs and chemicals, microangiopathic anaemia (p. 257), severe renal failure and severe liver disease. Burr cells are typical of renal failure.

Schistocytes
Red cell fragments. As for acanthocytes.

Changes in Intracellular Staining

Hypochromasia
Pale, lightly stained cells. Iron deficiency, thalassaemia, chronic systemic disease, lead poisoning, sideroblastic anaemia.

Polychromasia
Blue colour due to the presence of RNA in the cells, indicating immaturity. These cells are usually reticulocytes.

Anisochromasia (dimorphic film)
Two cell populations staining differently, usually one hypochromic and one not. Partly treated iron deficiency, multiple factor deficiency, sideroblastic anaemia, after blood transfusion.

Leptocytosis
Thin cells with a ring of haemoglobin and an unstained centre. Iron deficiency, thalassaemia and other haemoglobinopathies, liver disease, splenic removal or atrophy. They may be an artefact.

Target cells
Thin cells with central staining, an unstained inner ring and a stained outer ring. Causes as for leptocytosis.

Red Cell Inclusions

Punctate basophilia
Aggregated microsomes seen in haemolysis, erythrocyte regeneration after anaemia and lead poisoning.

Howell–Jolly bodies
Single small round basophilic bodies consisting of nuclear DNA remnants. Seen in splenic atrophy or removal, megaloblastic anaemia, haemolysis, leukaemia and any severe anaemia.

Heinz bodies
Denatured globin particles, seen as blue bodies in reticulocyte stains or recognized by special stains. Usually due to chemical poisoning and seen especially after splenectomy; also occur in glucose-6-phosphate dehydrogenase deficiency and rare haemoglobinopathies.

Siderocytes
Cells containing granules positive with iron stains, called Pappenheimer bodies. Caused by disturbed haem synthesis in lead poisoning, and sideroblastic anaemia; also after splenectomy and in haemolysis and haemochromatosis.

Reticulocytes
Young cells containing residual nuclear material which stains with cresyl blue. On standard films they cause macrocytosis and polychromasia.
   Normally 0.2–2.0% of cells are reticulocytes — but up to 4% in the newborn.
An increase is seen in:

1. Increased erythropoiesis — haemolysis (p. 253), bleeding and treatment of factor-deficiency anaemia.
2. Premature release from marrow — myelosclerosis, leuco-erythroblastic anaemia. Other immature cells are present.
3. Renal failure.

Nucleated red cells
These occur with intense marrow stimulation due to severe haemorrhage, haemolysis or hypoxia. They are also seen with pernicious anaemia, leukaemia, bone marrow infiltration and after splenectomy.

Miscellaneous

Rouleaux formation
Side-to-side adherence of cells in short columns. A non-specific phenomenon increased by high globulin and fibrinogen levels and associated with a high ESR.

Splenic disorders
After splenectomy, or in splenic atrophy due to infarction or steatorrhoea, target cells, schistocytes, Howell–Jolly bodies and a moderate leucocytosis and thrombocytosis appear. In hypersplenism there is anaemia, neutropenia, thrombocytopenia and a hyperplastic bone marrow.

Leucoerythroblastic anaemia
Cells normally confined to the marrow appear in the peripheral blood; nucleated red cells and myelocytes. It occurs with infiltration of the marrow by carcinoma and reticulosis, fibrosis, lipoid dystrophies or by tuberculosis. Secondary carcinoma is the commonest cause.

NUTRITIONAL-FACTOR DEFICIENCY ANAEMIA

Problems are seen mainly with iron and the vitamins B12 and folic acid.

Serum Iron

Normal

Adult males	9–29 μmol/l
Adult females	7–27 μmol/l
Neonates	18–45 μmol/l
Infants	7–18 μmol/l
Elderly	8–32 μmol/l
Pregnancy	a fall by about 35% to 6–30 μmol/l

The serum iron concentration is 25% lower at night than in the morning.

Increase
1. Iron overload — haemochromatosis (p. 136), haemosiderosis (p. 136), iron treatment and iron poisoning.
2. Contraceptive pill.
3. Cirrhosis.
4. Anaemia not due to iron deficiency — haemolysis, marrow hypoplasia, megaloblastic anaemia, sideroblastic anaemia.

Decrease
1. Iron deficiency.
2. Acute infection.
3. Chronic illness — infection, rheumatoid arthritis, malignancy.
4. Renal — nephrotic syndrome, uraemia.

Total Iron Binding Capacity (TIBC)
This measures the serum concentration of transferrin, the iron-carrying protein.

Normal

Adults	40–70 μmol/l
Infancy	20–60 μmol/l
Pregnancy	levels may almost double.

Increase
1. Iron deficiency.
2. Acute hepatitis.
3. Contraceptive pill.

Decrease
1. Iron overload — haemochromatosis and haemosiderosis.
2. Haemolysis.
3. Chronic disease — infection, cirrhosis, uraemia, cancer, rheumatoid disease.

Percentage Saturation of TIBC

Normal
Adults   20–40%
Neonates   higher
Pregnancy   lower

An increase is seen in conditions associated with a high serum iron, notably iron overload (p. 136). A decrease is characteristic of iron deficiency, but may be seen in acute infection.

Serum Ferritin

Normal
Adult males   15–200 μg/l
Adult females   12–150 μg/l
Infants   50–600 μg/l
Children   7–140 μg/l

Iron is stored in cells as ferritin, a complex of iron and the protein, apoferritin and as haemosiderin, aggregated ferritin. Serum ferritin is derived from the cells and is a measure of iron stores. It is, however, also raised in liver disease, chronic inflammatory and malignant disease.

Diagnosis of Iron-deficiency Anaemia
The typical picture is a hypochromic microcytic anaemia with a low serum iron, a high total iron-binding capacity (TIBC) and a TIBC saturation below 10%. In the mild case a low MCH and a rise in TIBC are early signs. Hypochromic anaemia with a low serum iron occurs in rheumatoid arthritis and other chronic diseases but as the TIBC is also low saturation is normal. Patients with thalassaemia and sideroblastic anaemia may have markedly hypochromic cells, but iron levels are normal. Iron deficiency may co-exist with these other hypochromic anaemias (except sideroblastic anaemia) and this can

be demonstrated by marked desaturation of the TIBC, absence of iron from the bone marrow, a reduced serum ferritin and a rise in haemoglobin with iron treatment. In a non-Caucasian it is wise to measure the serum ferritin or iron saturation before starting iron treatment, because of the possibility of thalassaemia.

Causes of Iron-deficiency Anaemia

1. Gastrointestinal blood loss — peptic ulcer, hiatus hernia, carcinoma, haemorrhoids, partial gastrectomy, salicylates.
2. Menstrual blood loss.
2. Dietary deficiency — especially in the elderly.
4. Pregnancy.
5. Malabsorption.

More than one cause may operate and frequently treatment is given on the basis of a provisional diagnosis, e.g. menorrhagia, without further investigation. Even in the absence of symptoms, gastrointestinal bleeding should be suspected if anaemia recurs after treatment, or fails to respond to it, if there is occult blood in the stools, a high ESR, or a leucocytosis. Hb rises about 1 g/dl per week and failure to respond may be due to tablets not taken, an ineffective slow release preparation, continued bleeding, malabsorption, or mis-diagnosis. Note that full investigation for bleeding is necessary in the male.

Serum Vitamin B12

Normal

Adults	140–700 ng/l (103–517 μmol/l)
Pregnancy	a fall by about 20%

The normal range depends greatly on the method used by the laboratory. Drugs, especially antibiotics and chemotherapeutic agents, interfere with bioassays and these are now being replaced by isotope techniques.

Vitamin B12 is found in animal products, combines with intrinsic factor secreted by the stomach, is absorbed in the ileum and is stored in the liver.

Increase
Liver disease and myeloproliferative disorder.

Decrease
1. Intrinsic factor deficiency — Addisonian pernicious anaemia (the commonest cause), partial and total gastrectomy.
2. Dietary deficiency — vegans, most often seen in Hindu women.
3. Ileal disease (p. 153).
4. Competition for the vitamin — bacterial contamination of the small bowel; the fish tapeworm.
5. Pregnancy — the vitamin B12 level is lower in megaloblastic anaemia of pregnancy than in normal preganancy, but the anaemia responds and vitamin B12 levels will usually rise with folate treatment alone.
6. Miscellaneous — in myxoedema and iron deficiency, vitamin B12 levels may be low in association with gastric mucosal atrophy. There is no megaloblastic change and Hb and vitamin B12 levels will rise with specific treatment.

Schilling Test

Normal
Over 10% of an oral dose appears in the urine in 24 hours. Absorption of vitamin B12 is measured by the urinary excretion of a small oral dose of radioactive vitamin flushed out by a large parenteral dose of unlabelled B12. Values below 5%, improved to normal when the test is repeated with oral intrinsic factor, suggest a gastric cause, usually Addisonian anaemia. Values between 5 and 10% occur in atrophic gastritis, malabsorption and occasionally in normals. Correction by a course of antibiotics suggests bacterial contamination of the gut. With ileal disease absorption is low and cannot be improved either by intrinsic factor or antibiotics. A Schilling test can be done after treatment with vitamin B12 has been started. A normal test does not completely rule out pernicious anaemia, as vitamin B12 in food may be less well absorbed.

Other Tests in Vitamin B12 Deficiency

Gastric parietal cell antibodies (GPCA)
These occur in over 70% of patients with pernicious anaemia and in up to 10% of other patients, especially older people, in autoimmune disease and atrophic gastritis. However, their association with megaloblastic anaemia is highly suggestive of pernicious anaemia.

Intrinsic factor antibodies
These are specific for pernicious anaemia, but are found in only 55% of patients. Sometimes they are present in gastric fluid when absent from the serum.

Gastric aspiration
Histamine-fast achlorhydria is invariable in pernicious anaemia, but it is not specific (p. 147).

Serum Folate

Normal
Adults	4.0–20.0 nmol/l
Pregnancy	2.0–10.0 nmol/l

Antibiotics interfere with the bioassay and the isotope methods are better. Low values commonly occur with mild or recent deficiency and the serum level is a poor guide to tissue stores, being low in up to one-third of hospital admissions.

Red Cell Folate

Normal
Whole blood in sequestrene tube

Adults	340–1020 nmol/l cells
Elderly	210–1130 nmol/l cells

It is the best guide to tissue stores, but may be low in uncomplicated vitamin B12 deficiency and may be misleadingly normal in megaloblastic anaemia of pregnancy, during a reticulocytosis, and after blood transfusion.

Folate Deficiency

Causes
1. Dietary deficiency — the commonest cause and often associated with pregnancy, old age, alcoholism and restricted diets.
2. Malabsorption — duodenal and jejunal disease (p. 153).
3. Increased demand — pregnancy, haemolysis, chronic infection, myeloproliferative disease.

4. Drugs — anticonvulsants, especially phenytoin but also barbiturates and primidone; antimetabolites, e.g. azathioprine and methotrexate; possibily also the contraceptive pill, PAS and co-trimoxazole.

Diagnosis of Megaloblastic Anaemia

Folic acid deficiency causes glossitis and megaloblastic anaemia, and vitamin B12 deficiency causes central and peripheral nervous system damage as well. Macrocytosis, polymorph hypersegmentation and pancytopenia are seen in the peripheral film and the finding of megaloblasts and giant metamyelocytes in the marrow is confirmatory. Raised serum unconjugated bilirubin, LDH and iron are the main biochemical changes. Iron deficiency or thalassaemia may mask the macrocytosis. Iron deficiency makes the marrow harder to interpret. In vitamin B12 deficiency the serum concentration is usually clearly low and folate levels are normal. Where Addisonian pernicious anaemia is not the cause serum antibodies are absent and the Schilling test is atypical. In folic acid deficiency severe enough to cause megaloblastic change, both serum and red cell folate levels are usually low, with the exceptions given above. Combined measurement of serum B12 and serum and red cell folate is usually sufficient to distinguish between folate and vitamin B12 deficiency. Folate measurements are misleading in pregnancy, but megaloblastic anaemia is nearly always due to folate deficiency in this circumstance.

Treatment with both folic acid and vitamin B12, never folic acid alone, can usually be started once levels of both vitamins and the sternal marrow have been taken. A reticulocyte response should occur by the sixth day of treatment, provided no other serious illness prevents it. When serum B12, folate and red cell folate levels are all low, the possibility of combined deficiency should be considered. Evaluation will include antibody tests, a Schilling test and a search for malabsorption. If doubt remains, a therapeutic trial with low-dose vitamin B12 (1 μg i.m. daily) may be undertaken first, followed, if necessary, by a trial with low-dose folic acid (200 μg/daily). If all vitamin levels are normal, possibilities include laboratory error, previous treatment and misdiagnosis. Alternative diagnoses are sideroblastic anaemia, erythroleukaemia, alcoholism and cytotoxic drugs.

HAEMOLYSIS

Anaemia occurs when increased red cell production cannot keep pace
with destruction. Haemolysis may be either or both intravascular or
extravascular, in which latter case cells are removed by the reticu-
loendothelial system. The first step is to demonstrate the presence of
haemolysis and then find its cause.

Causes of Haemolysis

Red cell defects
1. Haemoglobinopathies — thalassaemia, sickle-cell anaemia.
2. Congenital spherocytosis.
3. Glucose-6-phosphate dehydrogenase (G-6-PD) deficiency — drug
   precipitated.
4. Paroxysmal nocturnal haemoglobinuria.

Extracorpuscular agents
1. Isoimmune — transfusion reactions, rhesus incompatibility.
2. Autoimmune — Coombs' test is often positive
   (a) Idiopathic autoimmune haemolytic anaemia.
   (b) Infections — infectious mononucleosis, mycloplasma.
   (c) Systemic lupus erythematosus.
   (d) Malignancy — especially reticulosis and leukaemia.
   (e) Drugs — methyldopa, quinine, penicillin, cephalosporins.
3. Other drugs and poisons — phenacetin, sulphasalazine, benzene,
   heavy metals.
4. Other systemic disease — uraemia, liver disease, hypersplenism.
5. Other infection — malaria, septicaemia (DIC, p. 277).
6. Mechanical — microangiopathy, DIC, valvular prosthesis.

Evidence of Haemolysis
1. Abnormal red cells — spherocytes or schistocytes in the blood
   film.
2. Reticulocytosis — suggested by macrocytosis or polychromasia.
3. Bilirubin changes — serum unconjugated bilirubin raised, urine
   urobilinogen increased.
4. Evidence of intravascular haemolysis (p. 257).

5. Evidence of a specific haemolytic process or cell defect — Coombs' test, cold agglutinins, G-6-PD test.
6. Bone marrow activity increased.

TESTS FOR RED CELL DEFECTS

Osmotic Fragility Test

Normal
50% haemolysis occurs in a saline concentration of between 0.40 and 0.45%. Lysis occurring with stronger solutions is associated with spherocytosis, typically hereditary spherocytosis. It is not specific for this condition as spherocytosis is seen with other haemolytic diseases and the diagnosis is confirmed by the presence of abnormal fragility in relatives and the exclusion of other causes. The sensitivity of the test can be increased by prior incubation of the cells.

Glucose-6-Phosphate Dehydrogenase (G-6-PD) Deficiency
The enzyme G-6-PD maintains haemoglobin in the reduced state and deficiency, presents with acute haemolysis in response to infections, broad-bean ingestion (favism) and drugs, e.g. antimalarials, antibiotics, analgesics, quinidine and vitamin K. It occurs mainly in Asian, African and Mediterranean males (sex-linked recessive inheritance), rarely North Europeans. Heinz bodies may be seen in the blood film and 'in vitro' production of them is one screening test. Red cell G-6-PD can be measured by its effect on dye decolorization.

Haemoglobinopathies
The main haemoglobin of the adult red cell is HbA, comprising two α- and two β-polypeptide chains. Any change in these globin chains can critically affect the solubility of haemoglobin in the red cell or its capacity to combine reversibly with oxygen.

In thalassaemia the β-chains cannot be produced and fetal haemoglobin (HbF) with two α- and two γ-chains and HbA_2 with two α- and two δ-chains predominate. The homozygote presents in infancy with anaemia and jaundice. The heterozygote has a hypochromic anaemia in adult life. The condition occurs mainly in Asians and Mediterraneans.

Sickle-cell anaemia is due to a single abnormal amino acid in the β-chain. Homozygotes have over 80% HbS in their red cells and have severe anaemia with thrombotic crises owing to the rigidity of the sickle shaped red cells. Heterozygotes are liable to sickling under anoxic conditions. The condition occurs mainly in Africans. Other haemoglobin defects are less common.

Sickling Tests

Incubation of a sealed wet film causes sickling of red cells under reduced oxygen tension in the heterozygote, whereas it occurs in normal venous blood in the homozygote. This test is not as reliable as the solubility test, in which blood is centrifuged after dilution with a reducing agent. Sickle haemoglobin appears as a dark red surface band.

Alkali-denaturation Test

HbF is usually resistant to denaturation by alkali and this can be demonstrated in thalassaemia major and sickle-cell anaemia, where there is a significant amount of HbF, but not in thalassaemia trait.

Haemoglobin Electrophoresis

This is necessary for diagnosis of heterozygotes with sickle-cell trait, thalassaemia minor, mixed haemoglobinopathies, and rare haemoglobins. In normal adults there is less than 3% HbA_2 and less than 1% HbF, though rather more HbF in children under four years. Increased amounts are found in thalassaemia and sickle-cell anaemia where HbS also occurs.

TESTS FOR EXTRACORPUSCULAR AGENTS

Haemolysis is often part of a systemic illness. The tests below are indicated.

Coombs' Test (Antiglobulin Test)

Red cells sensitized by a coating of antibody globulin are agglutinated by serum containing an antibody against human globulin (AHG). The AHG serum is raised from an animal immunized against human globulin. In the direct test, antibody coating the patient's red cells is detected by agglutinating them with AHG after first washing them with saline to remove serum. The indirect test detects antibody free in the serum. The patient's serum is incubated with compatible red cells. These cells, now coated with antibody, are washed and treated with AHG as for the direct Coombs' test. Both direct and indirect tests are carried out and different globulin and complement components coating the cell can be detected. Autoimmune haemolytic anaemia (AIHA) is the commonest cause of a positive test, but the test may be positive without haemolysis.

Positive Coombs' test
1. Autoimmune haemolytic anaemia (warm reactive). IgG autoantibodies coat the red cell surface. AIHA may be idiopathic or associated with systemic lupus erythematosus, lymphoma, leukaemia or carcinoma.
2. Autoimmune haemolytic anaemia (cold reactive). IgM antibodies coat the cell, often transiently. AIHA may occur as a primary event or follow infectious mononucleosis or mycoplasma pneumonia.
3. Drugs — antibodies to drugs, e.g. methyldopa, attach to drug molecules, coating the cell and activate complement.
4. Alloantibodies — the commonest example of this is haemolytic disease of the newborn, in which maternal IgG coats the fetal cells.

Cold Agglutinins
Normal titre up to 1:32.
Group O red cells are directly agglutinated by serial dilutions of the patient's serum at 4°C, but not at room temperature. The blood must be kept at 37°C until the test is started.
They are found in high titre sometimes in normal persons and in pregnancy and are of not much diagnostic help. Titres over 1:1000 may be associated with haemolysis.

Postive test
1. Haemolytic anaemia — Coombs' test positive.
2. Paroxysmal cold haemoglobinuria — a modification of the test, the Donath–Landsteiner reaction, is used.
3. Infections — mycoplasma pneumonia, malaria, infectious mononucleosis, adenovirus, influenza.
4. Miscellaneous — cirrhosis, leukaemia, myeloma.

Causes of Intravascular Haemolysis
1. Incompatible transfusion.
2. Drugs, chemicals and toxins.
3. Infections.
4. Microangiopathic haemolytic anaemia. There is fragmentation of red cells and sometimes DIC (p. 277). It is seen with haemolytic uraemic syndrome, malignant hypertension, pre-eclamptic tox- aemia, vasculitis and thrombotic thrombocytopenic purpura. Damage to the red blood cells is caused by abnormality in small blood vessels. In haemolytic uraemic syndrome there is also an acute nephritis. In thrombotic thrombocytopenic purpura there is nephritis, thrombocytopenia and cerebral damage.
5. Chronic intravascular haemolysis — this occurs in paroxysmal nocturnal haemoglobinuria and haemolysis associated with cold agglutinins.

Evidence of Intravascular Haemolysis
When haemolysis occurs in the blood stream the plasma haemoglo- bin level rises and the free haemoglobin combines with haptoglobin, the complex being metabolized so that the haptoglobin level falls. When the haptoglobin is used up, haemoglobin combines with albumin to form methaemalbumin and appears in the urine as free haemoglobin.

Serum Haptoglobin

Normal
Clotted blood: haemolysis must be avoided.

Adults	0.30–2.0 g/l, slightly lower in females than males
Neonates	0.00–2.0 g/l

It is measured by the capacity of serum to bind haemoglobin. An increase is seen in many severe systemic diseases, but a decrease to below 0.1 g/l suggests intravascular or severe extravascular haemoly- sis, in the absence of chronic liver disease. A decrease due to haemolysis might be masked by a rise due to the simultaneous presence of systemic disease.

Plasma Haemoglobin

Normal
Whole blood in a sequestrene tube.

10–40 mg/l (0.16–0.62 μmol/l)

A large rise occurs in intravascular haemolysis and a small rise sometimes in severe haemoglobinopathies and autoimmune haemolysis. Slight rises are often due to haemolysis of the blood during collection.

Plasma Methaemalbumin
This is normally absent when centrifuged plasma obtained from heparinized whole blood is examined by spectroscopy. The sensitivity of the test may be increased by prior conversion to an ammonium pigment (Schumm's test). Its presence is diagnostic of severe intravascular haemolysis, occurring otherwise only sometimes in severe acute pancreatitis.

Urine Haemoglobin
This is distinguished from haematuria by the absence of red cells in the sediment and the presence of pigment in the supernatant is confirmed by spectroscopy or a dipstick test.

Urine Haemosiderin
In chronic haemoglobinaemias, especially paroxysmal nocturnal haemoglobinuria (PNH), the sediment contains haemosiderin granules, derived from haemoglobin, which stain blue with Perl's ferrocyanide test. This is a good sign of chronic intravascular haemolysis.

Acid Lysis Test (Ham)
The patient's red cells haemolyze rapidly on incubation in acidified normal serum. The test is positive in PNH, but weak positives occur in other conditions.

MARROW FAILURE

The bone marrow is hypoplastic on examination. Iron is usually increased in stores but absent from red cell precursors.

Causes

1. Marrow replacement — neoplasm, leukaemia, fibrosis.
2. Idiopathic aplastic anaemia.
3. Systemic disease — renal failure, neoplasms, infection, rheumatoid disease, liver disease, hypothyroidism.
4. Drug induced.
   (a) Dose related — irradiation and antineoplastic agents.
   (b) Idiosyncratic.

The drugs given below are relatively high risk, but many others may be responsible. Red cells, white cells, or platelets may be selectively affected. Drugs taken without the knowledge of the physician may be responsible.

Antibiotics	chloramphenicol, sulphonamides.
Anticonvulsants	hydantoins, trimethadione, paramethadione.
Antirheumatics	phenylbutazone, gold, indomethacin, aspirin.
Antithyroid agents	potassium perchlorate, carbimazole.
Others	phenothiazines, benzothiadiazines, frusemide, quinidine, chlorpropamide.

BLOOD VOLUME MEASUREMENTS

Red cell volume is measured by radiochromium in the study of polycythaemia. More rapid methods are useful in the control of acute surgical shock and bleeding abdominal aneurysms.

Red cell volume
Adult males   28–33 ml/kg
Adult females   23–30 ml/kg

Plasma volume
40–50 ml/kg

Whole blood volume
65–85 ml/kg

Polycythaemia
This is best assessed and treated using haematocrit levels measured directly by centrifugation. Levels of 55% in males and 50% in females are diagnostic. A red cell count may be necessary to confirm an increase in cells where haemoglobin content is reduced by iron

deficiency. Red cell volume measurement is necessary to make a firm diagnosis of polycythaemia rubra vera (PRV).

Causes
1. Relative polycythaemia — red cell volume is normal but plasma volume is low. Seen in fluid depletion (p. 30) and 'stress' pseudopolycythaemia of middle-aged men.
2. Secondary polycythaemia — red cell volume is high but there are no other features of PRV. Increased erythropoietin secretion occurs. The usual cause is hypoxia, but it is seen rarely in renal disease, carcinoma, cysts, ischaemia and hydronephrosis, and also with tumours of the liver and cerebellum.
3. Polycythaemia rubra vera (PRV) — this is a myeloproliferative disorder characterized by erythrocytosis, leucocytosis, thrombocytosis and a raised leucocyte alkaline phosphatase and splenomegaly. There is a tendency to arterial and venous thrombosis and abnormal bleeding.

ERYTHROCYTE SEDIMENTATION RATE (ESR) (WESTERGREN)

Normal
Whole blood in sodium citrate bottle (2.5 ml)

Adult males	0–15 mm/l per h
Adult females	0–20 mm/l per h
Children	0–10 mm/l per h
Over 50 years (males)	0–20 mm/l per h
(females)	0–30 mm/l per h
Pregnancy	30–95 mm/l per h

Sedimentation is rapid when red cells form rouleaux in response to increased fibrinogen and globulin levels. It is a very useful but non-specific test used to screen for systemic disease and monitor its progress. Unexpected results should be repeated.

Limitations of the ESR
1. Technical — false low values are seen if too much anticoagulant is used or if the blood stands for more than two hours before measurement, and false high values if the tube is tilted.

2. Unexpected normal values — these can occur in many systemic diseases, for example fibrotic neoplasms, and even in widely disseminated malignant disease.
3. Unexpected high values — these give no clue to the nature of any disease present and excessive investigation in the absence of other evidence of illness might be unhelpful. Equally, a high ESR could be a sign of an occult tuberculosis.

Decrease in ESR
Levels may be low in polycythaemia, heart failure, plasma protein deficiency, sickle-cell anaemia, cryoglobulinaemia and corticosteroid treatment. This is of importance in that it may mask an elevation due to other causes.

Diseases often associated with a normal ESR
1. Infections confined to the blood stream, e.g. bacteraemia, or epithelial surfaces, e.g. cystitis.
2. Viral illnesses, e.g. infectious mononucleosis.
3. CNS disease.

Increase in ESR
1. Inflammation of any kind is a common cause.
2. Tissue infarction, e.g. myocardial infarction.
3. Dysproteinaemia — abnormal globulins in neoplastic and immunological disease, e.g. cold agglutinins, glomerular disease and liver disease.
4. Drugs — oestrogens, contraceptive pill.

Markedly increased ESR (over 100 mm/l per h)
1. Malignancy — especially of blood or bone.
2. Connective tissue diseases (Chap. 14) and systemic vasculitis.
3. Renal disease, especially nephrotic syndrome.
4. Infections such as miliary tuberculosis and kala-azar. Pneumonia in elderly people is a common reversible cause.
5. Sarcoidosis.

The progress of disease may be monitored by the ESR level, though it may remain elevated due to persistent plasma protein abnormalities even though the disease is inactive. The C-reactive protein can be helpful in this case.

ESR as a specific test
Certain diseases are always associated with a high ESR and the test is most useful in the diagnosis of polymyalgia rheumatica (p. 144) and temporal arteritis. A normal ESR is also important evidence against any active vasculitis or haematological malignancy.

Chapter Twenty Three

DISEASES OF THE WHITE BLOOD CELLS

The main function of white blood cells is in defence against infection. Neutrophil granulocytes and monocytes act by phagocytosis. Lymphocytes and plasma cells are concerned with antibody production. Basophil and eosinophil granulocytes are particularly involved in allergic and autoimmune disease. Neutrophils, basophils and eosinophils are produced entirely in the bone marrow. Lymphocytes, monocytes and plasma cells are derived mainly from lymphoid tissue.

Total White Blood Cell Count (WBC)

Normal
Whole blood 5 ml in sequestrene tube for total and differential count.

Adults	$4.0–11.0 \times 10^9/l$
Neonates	$9.0–30.0 \times 10^9/l$
Infants	$5.0–19.0 \times 10^9/l$
Children	$4.5–15.5 \times 10^9/l$
Elderly	$3.1– 8.9 \times 10^9/l$
Pregnancy	
(1st trimester)	$3.1–15.3 \times 10^9/l$
(2nd and 3rd	
trimesters)	$5.0–16.6 \times 10^9/l$
(post partum)	$20.0 \quad \times 10^9/l$

Nucleated red cells are included in the white cell count by electronic counters.

Neutrophil Leucocytes

Normal

Adults	$2.7-7.5 \times 10^9/l$ (40–75% of total WBC)
Neonates	35–60% dropping to infant levels in a few days
Infants	30–50% ⎫ differential counts may be mis-
Children	30–65% ⎭ leading
Elderly	$1.8-6.5 \times 10^9/l$
Pregnancy	The increase in total WBC is largely due to neutrophil leucocytes

Increase (neutrophil leucocytosis)
1. Infection — usually bacterial and counts $> 30.0 \times 10^9/l$ suggest abscess formation.
2. Tissue destruction — trauma, burns, infarctions, neoplasms.
3. Blood loss — haemorrhage and haemolysis.
4. Metabolic disorder — acidosis, uraemia, acute gout, after exertion and convulsions.
5. Drug induced — corticosteroids, poisons, contraceptive pill.
6. Myeloproliferative disease.

Decrease (neutropenia)
1. Infection — especially viral, such as influenza, hepatitis and infectious mononucleosis. Also overwhelming bacterial infection, typhoid, brucellosis and malaria.
2. Bone marrow depression (p. 258).
3. Factor deficiency anaemia — usually vitamin B12 and folate, but occasionally iron.
4. Hypersplenism.
5. Systemic lupus erythematosus.
6. Leukaemia.

Effects of neutropenia
Fatigue and sensitivity to infection, especially of the throat, will usually appear at counts below $0.5 \times 10^9/l$. Gram-negative septicaemia is a particular danger.

Neutrophil Abnormalities

'Left' shift
There is a majority of immature cells with two or less nuclear lobes. This is seen with infection, toxaemia, leukaemia and leucoerythroblastic anaemia (p. 246). In the latter two cases even less mature forms, such as metamyelocytes, are likely to be seen.

'Right' shift
There is a majority of older cells with four or more nuclear lobes. This is seen in folic acid and vitamin B12 deficiency, renal failure, liver disease, rheumatoid arthritis, sometimes in sepsis and iron deficiency, and rarely in normal people.

Toxic granulation
Purple granules with standard haematological stains are seen in severe infection and markedly toxic conditions. Toxic granulations also occur with pre-eclampsia and after radiotherapy.

Leucocyte Alkaline Phosphatase (LAP)
Normal score 15–100: fingerprick specimen
One hundred consecutive neutrophils are graded 0–4, according to the intensity of staining with a reagent that colours the alkaline phosphatase granules. A marked increase is typical of polycythaemia rubra vera (PRV) and leukaemoid reactions. A moderate increase may be seen with pregnancy, oestrogens, neutrophilia of any cause, secondary polycythaemia, and some patients with myeloproliferative syndromes other than PRV.

A decrease is seen in chronic myelocytic leukaemia (CML) and paroxysmal nocturnal haemoglobinuria (PNH).

The test is useful in the diagnosis of PRV, PNH and CML. CML may be difficult to recognize in the aleukaemic phase or difficult to differentiate from a leukaemoid reaction or other forms of myeloproliferative disorder. In CML, the LAP is low and the Philadelphia chromosome is often present.

Eosinophils

Normal
$0.04–0.45 \times 10^9/l$ (1–6%)

Increase (eosinophilia)
This often indicates the presence of a foreign protein or other allergen.

1. Allergy — asthma, hay fever, serum sickness, urticaria, drugs and food sensitivity. Counts usually below $1.0 \times 10^9/l$. Drug allergy is a common cause and there may be no other reaction. Penicillins are common offenders.
2. Infestations — with tissue invasion by parasites counts may reach $15 \times 10^9/l$. It may occur in malaria.
3. Associated with pulmonary infiltration.
   (a) Tropical — filariasis.
   (b) Temperate zone — cough and infiltrations lasting for a few weeks, sometimes called Löffler's syndrome. Caused by helminths such as *Ascaris*, drugs such as nitrofurantoin or idiopathic. A chronic eosinophilic pneumonia lasting for months also occurs.
   (c) Asthmatic — usually due to aspergillosis (p. 86).
   (d) Vasculitis — polyarteritis, etc; eosinophilia may be marked.
4. Infections — convalescent phase.
5. Skin disease — usually extensive but not necessarily allergic.
6. Miscellaneous — reticulosis, sarcoidosis, myeloproliferative disorders and leukaemia.

Eosinopenia is seen in Cushing's disease, steroid treatment and acute illness.

Basophils

Normal
$0–0.1 \times 10^9/l$ (0–1%)

Basophilia is commonest in chronic myeloid leukaemia and can occur in all myeloproliferative disorders and malignancy.

Lymphocytes

Normal

Adults	$1.5–3.5 \times 10^9/l$ (20–45% of total WBC)
Neonates	$< 12.0 \times 10^9/l$
Infants	$< 60\%$ total WBC

Children   < 50% total WBC
Elderly $0.7–3.5 \times 10^9/l$

Increase (lymphocytosis)
1. Infection in children — this commonly occurs instead of a neutrophil leucocytosis.
2. Viral infection — exanthemata, influenza, hepatitis, infectious mononucleosis and infectious lymphocytosis.
3. Bacterial infection — pertussis causes especially high counts; tuberculosis, syphilis, typhoid, brucellosis.
4. Convalescent phase of any infection.
5. Lymphocytic leukaemia and reticulosis.

A decreased count is found with steroid treatment, Cushing's disease and protein-calorie malnutrition.

Atypical lymphocytes
In viral infections, 'virocytes', larger cells with darker blue staining cytoplasm, may be seen. Large cells with characteristic abundant pale blue cytoplasm are seen in infectious mononucleosis, toxoplasmosis and cytomegalovirus infections.

Monocytes

Normal
$0.2–0.8 \times 10^9/l$ (2–10%)

Increase
1. Bacterial infection — tuberculosis, brucellosis, typhoid, bacterial endocarditis, convalescence from acute infection.
2. Protozoal infections — malaria, trypanosomiasis.
3. Malignancy — myeloma, monocytic leukaemia, lymphadenoma.
4. Chronic diseases — connective-tissue disease, ulcerative colitis, Crohn's disease.

Leukaemoid Reaction
This is a marked elevation of the total white cell count, usually over $50 \times 10^9/l$ with circulating immature cells. It resembles leukaemia, but the haemoglobin and platelets are normal and the leucocyte alkaline phosphatase is raised. The bone marrow is diagnostic. It

occurs in response to severe infection, especially in children, in tuberculosis, malignancy and acute haemolysis. The cells are usually of the myeloid series, but in pertussis and infectious mononucleosis they are lymphocytes and in rubella they may be plasma cells.

Leukaemia

Acute leukaemias begin abruptly with fatigue and fever. There is anaemia and thrombocytopenia. Peripheral white cell counts vary, but the cells are always immature and abnormal. The marrow is overrun by blast cells. Acute lymphoblastic leukaemia (ALL) occurs in children and older people. A surface membrane marker is found on the cells. Acute myeloblastic leukaemia (AML) occurs in young adults. Leucocyte alkaline phosphatase (LAP) is absent.

In chronic myelocytic leukaemia (CML) the spleen is always enlarged. Neutrophil granulocytes proliferate in the blood and bone marrow. LAP is usually low. The Philadelphia chromosome is found in cultured myeloid cells. Chronic lymphocytic leukaemia (CLL) is associated with large numbers of circulating mature lymphocytes which also eventually overrun and suppress the marrow. Immuno-globulin levels may be low and the direct antiglobulin test may be positive (p. 255).

Chapter Twenty Four

DISORDERS OF HAEMOSTASIS

The functions of the haemostatic system are to confine the blood to the vascular bed, maintain the patency of that bed and stop bleeding from injured vessels. Bleeding is arrested by contraction of the vessel walls, formation of a platelet plug and, lastly, by formation of a fibrin clot. Abnormal bleeding is caused by a defect in the vessels, the platelets, or the coagulation mechanism.

Clinical Problems
The haemostatic mechanism is investigated in the following circumstances.
1. Systemic disease — there may be a condition such as hepatic or renal failure known to be associated with abnormal bleeding. Bleeding in the course of acute illness may suggest disseminated intravascular coagulation (DIC).
2. Abnormal bleeding without obvious systemic disease — there is bleeding without sufficient local cause. Commonly there is purpura or bruising.
3. Hereditary predisposition — investigation of an infant from a family affected by a bleeding disorder may be necessary.
4. Organ biopsy — the safety of this must be demonstrated beforehand.

Screening Tests
An accurate history of previous bleeding, a family history and a drug history are taken. A blood film, platelet count, activated partial thromboplastin time, prothrombin time, and thrombin time are necessary. A bleeding time is required if a vascular or platelet abnormality is suspected.

Vascular Defects
These cause skin bleeding and melaena, rarely generalized bleeding.

Local pressure is effective in stopping bleeding. The bleeding time may be abnormal but tests are not very satisfactory.

Causes
1. Vasculitis — systemic necrotizing vasculitis; Henoch-Schönlein disease; septicaemia, e.g. meningococcal; drug induced, e.g. warfarin, thiazides, sulphonamide; dysproteinaemias (p. 18). The lesions may be palpable in vasculitis.
2. Connective-tissue defects — purpura simplex or easy bruising seen in women; senile purpura; steroid purpura; scurvy; hereditary disorders, e.g. pseudoxanthoma elasticum.
3. Miscellaneous — vascular dilatations, childhood exanthemata, fat embolism.

Platelet Disorders
There may be thrombocytopenia or a qualitative platelet disorder. Bleeding occurs into the skin and the brain and from mucous membranes usually immediately after trauma. Bleeding is common at counts below $40 \times 10^9/l$ and at counts below $10 \times 10^9/l$ it is usual and often severe.

Investigation
The bleeding time is prolonged but the test is unnecessary in thrombocytopenia. Clot retraction is abnormal in thrombocytopenia and also in thrombasthenia. Bone marrow examination is necessary in thrombocytopenia to study megakaryocyte numbers and morphology. Abnormal platelet may be inferred from the study of platelet morphology and platelet aggregation tests.

Platelet Count

Normal
Whole blood in a sequestrene tube

Adults	$150–400 \times 10^9/l$
Neonates	$90–480 \times 10^9/l$ (adult levels after the first week)

In adults one platelet is seen for every 10–20 red cells in a stained blood film.

Increase (thrombocytosis)
1. Neoplastic disease — carcinoma, myeloproliferative disorder and reticulosis.
2. Severe illness — trauma (including surgery), infection, inflammation.
3. Rebound thrombocytosis — recovery from haemorrhage, haemolysis, pernicious anaemia, alcoholism, and after splenectomy.

Decrease (thrombocytopenia)
1. Reduction of megakaryocytes — this is seen in marrow infiltration and hypoplasia of all causes (p. 258), e.g. myelofibrosis, or drugs, including alcohol.
2. Ineffective thrombocytopoiesis — this is most often seen in megaloblastic anaemia but can occur in leukaemia. Megakaryocytes may be normal or increased.
3. Reduced platelet survival — there is increased destruction induced by drugs or associated with autoimmune thrombocytopenic purpuras. Increased platelet consumption occurs in acute infections, such as septicaemia or malaria, thrombotic thrombocytopenic purpura, haemolytic-uraemic syndrome and disseminated intravascular coagulation.
4. Sequestration of platelets — hypersplenism.

Qualitative platelet defects
These should be suspected when the platelet count is normal but abnormality is found in the bleeding time or platelet morphology.

Causes
1. Congenital — von Willebrand's disease, hereditary thrombasthenia.
2. Drug induced — aspirin, dipyridamole, antihistamines, dextran infusion, non-steroidal anti-inflammatory drugs.
3. Haematological malignancy — sometimes an early sign, e.g. acute leukaemia.
4. Miscellaneous — renal failure, scurvy, thrombocythaemia, γ-globulin abnormalities.

Bleeding time
Normal — 2–9 min.

With the Ivy method, a cuff is put round the upper arm at 40 mmHg and three punctures are made in the forearm, with a spring lancet. Blood is soaked up with filter paper.

The bleeding time is abnormal, particularly in platelet disorders but also with vascular defects. It is useful in the detection of qualitative platelet disorders, especially those caused by drugs such as aspirin. It may be abnormal in von Willebrand's disease, but is not usually so in classical haemophilia.

The Clotting Mechanism

The clotting process is a chain reaction which progressively increases in rate as each factor is activated in turn. It can be initiated by the intrinsic system, involving only blood components, or by the extrinsic system, involving tissue factors. These converge to a common path (Figure 24.1). This sequential process, with magnification allows the process to be inhibited during its course and the amount of clot produced to be controlled.

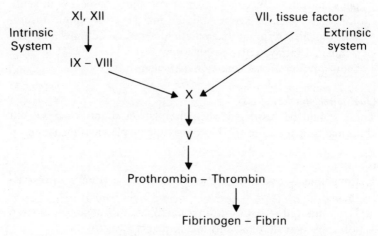

Figure 24.1 The clotting chain.

Bleeding may occur when any of the components are defective, inhibited, or used up by disseminated intravascular coagulation. A clotting tendency occurs locally when blood flow is slowed and generally when a coagulant enters the circulation or a natural anticoagulant, such as antithrombin, is lost.

Coagulation Defects
There is spontaneous bleeding into joints, muscles and viscera. After minor trauma there may be a delay, followed by persistent oozing; local pressure does not stop the bleeding.

Causes
1. Liver disease — bleeding is usually from peptic ulcer or varices. (Factors I, II, V, VII, IX, and X may be deficient).
2. Vitamin K deficiency — occurs in the newborn and in malabsorption, especially biliary obstruction. It is less common with other types of malabsorption, but may be seen after antibiotics, when dietary deficiency may be contributory. It is a feature of oral anticoagulation. There is impaired production of factors II, VII, IX and X.
3. Disseminated intravascular coagulation (DIC) (see p. 277).
4. Congenital deficiencies — the commonest are factor VIII (haemophilia, von Willebrand's disease) and factor IX (Christmas disease). There is usually a family history and they are commoner in males.

Investigation of Clotting Defects
The major coagulation factors are listed in Table 24.1. The prothrombin time (PT) tests the extrinsic system and the activated partial thromboplastin time (APTT) tests the intrinsic system. If only one of these is abnormal, then factors in the other pathway and the final common path are normal. If both are abnormal, then there is either a defect in the final path or there are multiple problems. If the test is corrected by adding the specific factor or by plasma missing a different factor, e.g. from a patient with haemophilia, there is probably a factor deficiency. A slow inibitor might be present and this is detected by a progressive inactivation test. If mixing with the deficient factor does not normalize the test, an inactivator, either an antibody or an inhibitor, such as heparin, is present. The formation of the fibrin clot and its stabilization are tested by the thrombin clotting time and a clot solubility test.

Whole Blood Clotting Time

Normal
5–11 min.

Table 24.1 Coagulation Factors

Factor	Synonym	Tests for deficiency
I	Fibrinogen	BT, PT, APTT, TCT
II	Prothrombin	PT, APTT
III	Thromboplastin	
IV	Calcium	
V	Proaccelerin	PT, APTT
VII	Proconvertin	PT
VIII	Antihaemophilic globulin (AHG)	APTT
IX	Christmas factor (PTC)	APTT
X	Stuart-Prower factor	PT, APTT
XI	Plasma thromboplastin antecedent (PTA)	APTT
XII	Hageman factor	APTT
XIII	Fibrin stabilizing factor	

BT   = bleeding time
PT   = prothrombin time
APTT = activated partial thromboplastin time
TCT = thrombin clotting time

Venous blood in a glass tube is put in a water bath at 37°C and tilted every thirty seconds until clotting occurs. This is a simple but not very sensitive and accurate screening test most useful for detecting defects of the intrinsic system.

Activated Partial Thromboplastin Time (Kaolin Cephalin Time, APTT)

Normal
Citrated whole blood.
35–50 s (according to method used)

This is the time taken for citrated plasma to clot in the presence of kaolin (factor XII activator), cephalin (platelet substitute) and calcium. If the prothrombin time is normal, an abnormal test usually indicates deficiency of factors VIII or IX, occasionally of XII or XI. It is a sensitive reliable test of the intrinsic system. The exact deficiency can be determined by normalization of the clotting time with the addition of plasma specifically deficient in only one of the factors under study.

Prothrombin Time (One Stage, Quick)

Normal
Citrated whole blood.
11–18 s (according to method used)

Usually expressed as a ratio to a normal control.

This is the time taken for a mixture of calcium, citrated plasma and tissue thromboplastin to clot. It tests the extrinsic system, bypassing the intrinsic system, and is sensitive to deficiency of factors VII, X, V, II and I. It is abnormal in vitamin K deficiency, liver disease and DIC. It is also prolonged by treatment with heparin and oral anticoagulants.

A two-stage test, more sensitive to prothrombin deficiency but unaffected by deficiency of the earlier factors in the cascade, is available.

Thrombin Clotting Time (TCT)

Normal
Citrated whole blood.
9–13 s

When thrombin is added to citrated plasma the clot should form within 3 s of the control and be of good quality.

Abnormality occurs with fibrinogen deficiency, abnormal fibrinogen or inhibition of conversion of fibrinogen to fibrin by heparin or fibrin degeneration products. It is seen in liver failure and intravascular clotting. Circulating inhibitors of clotting can occur in SLE, postpartum and haemophilia. In this case the TCT of normal plasma is prolonged if the patient's plasma is added to it.

Plasma Fibrinogen

Normal
Citrated whole blood.
1.5–4.0 g/l

The quantity of fibrin that can be precipitated from plasma is measured by its turbidity. A rapid test for severe fibrinogen deficiency is the 'fibrinogen titre', in which thrombin is added to serial dilutions of plasma. Visible clot is normally seen down to dilutions of 1:128.

Increase
1. Pregnancy and oestrogen treatment.
2. Acute tissue damage or infection.
3. Nephrotic syndrome.
4. Collagen disease — proportional to disease activity in rheumatoid arthritis and rheumatic carditis.

Decrease
This occurs particularly in DIC, but also in severe liver disease, as it is made in the liver. A mild decrease occurs in many diseases.

Fibrin Degradation Products (FDP)
Whole blood in special tube containing thrombin and proteolytic inhibitor.

Normal
< 10 mg/l

These can be measured by the agglutination of latex particules coated with antibody to FDP. Increased FDPs are evidence of increased fibrinolysis and therefore usually of intravascular fibrin deposition. They are found in venous thrombosis, pulmonary embolism, DIC and recent myocardial infarction. They also occur with menstruation, hepatic cirrhosis and renal failure.

Clot Retraction
Whole blood, not anticoagulated.
When venous blood is kept in a glass tube in a water bath at 37°C it retracts to about half its volume, forming a firm rubbery clot, within an hour. Abnormality is seen in thrombocytopenia, thrombasthenia and hypofibrinogenaemia. Thrombocytosis and hyperfibrinogenaemia also impede clot retraction.

FIBRINOLYSIS

The clotting chain is in balance with the fibrinolytic system. Circulating plasminogen is activated to plasmin, which breaks down fibrinogen and fibrin clots, releasing fibrin degradation products.

Disseminated Intravascular Coagulation (DIC)
Also called consumption coagulopathy and defibrination syndrome. Activation of the clotting system causes fibrin deposition, exhausts haemostatic factors and stimulates fibrinolysis, and intravascular destruction of red cells and platelets may occur. There is usually bleeding into the skin, from the gut, and from venepuncture sites. Thrombosis may occur. Renal, hepatic, cardiac, or respiratory failure are associated with DIC or its cause. There is thrombocytopenia, reduced serum fibrinogen, increased FDP, prolonged TCT, abnormal PT and APTT and abnormal whole blood clotting. There may be evidence of microangiopathic haemolysis (p. 257).

Causes
1. Obstetric complications.
2. Infection — Gram-negative, *Staph. aureus*, meningococcal septicaemia, cerebral malaria, gas gangrene.
3. Malignancy — leukaemia, prostatic carcinoma.
4. Severe trauma — accidental or surgical.
5. Mismatched blood transfusion.
6. Heat stroke.
7. Anaphylactic shock.

CONTROL OF THERAPEUTIC ANTICOAGULATION

With continuous heparin infusion the partial thromboplastin time should be kept at 2–2.5 times the normal control or the whole blood clotting time should be prolonged to 20–30 minutes. A check should be made 6 hours after starting treatment, then daily. With intermittent heparin injections tests should be taken 30 minutes before the next dose.

Oral anticoagulants are controlled by the one-stage prothrombin time (PT), measured twice weekly for the first two weeks. According to clinical judgement the PT should be prolonged 2–3 times the control value.

Chapter Twenty Five

DRUGS AND POISONS

Therapeutic Levels

The measurement of plasma drug levels has a limited role in the control of treatment. The estimations are sometimes difficult. They indicate the total level, including protein-bound drug, and not the biologically active free level. They do not indicate drug concentration in the target tissue. Also, various factors, such as other drugs given, the patient's condition, and fluid and electrolyte disturbances, as well as the plasma levels, affect toxicity and therapeutic effectiveness. It is usual therefore to assess the dose of a drug by the age, sex, and weight of a patient. Doses are reduced if there is liver damage and the drug is metabolized by the liver, or if there is renal damage and the drug or its toxic metabolites are excreted by the kidney. The serum creatinine provides an estimate of renal function. Dose size may be reduced to avoid peak levels with short-acting drugs and dose intervals may be increased to avoid accumulation of the drug.

Plasma drug levels are most helpful where there is a narrow margin between the therapeutic and toxic dose and where the same dose can produce markedly different plasma concentrations in different patients. It is important that blood be taken at the correct time in relation to drug administration, particularly with drugs that have a short half-life. The best guide to drug treatment will always be the old maxim that few drugs should be used and they should be known well.

Poisoning

Sometimes unknown poisons can be identified and blood levels can also be determined. However, many factors affect the management of the poisoned patient, including general condition, other drugs taken, whether blood levels are rising or falling, and the time which has elapsed since the poisoning.

Digoxin

Clotted blood or heparinized plasma collected at least 12 hours after the last dose, with the patient preferably on the same dose for a week. Therapeutic range 1.0–2.0 μg/l (1.2–2.6 μmol/l).

Children are more resistant to toxicity than adults.

Digoxin is measured by a radioimmunoassay with which spironolactone interferes. A level of below 1.0 μg/l makes toxicity unlikely and above 2.0 μg/l it becomes increasingly probable. At a given level, the probability of toxicity is increased by hypokalaemia, hypocalcaemia, hypoxia, hypothyroidism, sympathetic overactivity, and severe myocardial disease. The opposite states are protective. These factors, as well as the serum level, must be considered when possible toxicity is assessed. Hypoxia and hypokalaemia are particularly important. Toxicity manifests usually with nausea or disturbance of cardiac rhythm. ST segment depression on the ECG (p. 199) indicates digitalis effect, not necessarily toxicity. In the absence of digoxin levels, dosage is adjusted according to the serum creatinine level, age and weight. In atrial fibrillation, where the drug is most clearly indicated, the resting heart rate is controlled to about 80/min. Average daily maintenance doses for a male and female are 0.325 and 0.25 mg respectively, but there is considerable variation.

Antibiotics

In general, the adequacy of treatment is checked by the therapeutic response. In subacute bacterial endocarditis the patient's serum should be bactericidal against the infecting organism at a dilution of at least 1:4. The avoidance of toxicity is especially important with the aminoglycosides.

Aminoglycoside antibiotics

The dose of gentamicin given depends on the patient's size, and the dose interval on renal function. Persistent high levels are more dangerous than intermittent peaks. The peak level should be between 6 and 12 μg/ml one hour after i.m. or half an hour after i.v. injection. Trough levels before the next injection should be below 2 μg/ml. The minimum required concentration also depends on the sensitivity of the infecting organism. An average dose level is 80 mg eight-hourly, but it is always best to measure blood levels to avoid ototoxicity and nephrotoxicity. The dangers are increased with prolonged treatment, ECF depletion, renal impairment and concurrent use of loop diuretics or cephalosporins. Levels are similar for tobramycin, but higher for amikacin.

Anticonvulsants

Therapeutic levels
Clotted blood or heparinized plasma collected at the trough point. Phenytoin 10–20 mg/l (40–80 μmol/l). Ataxia appears at about 30 mg/l. The average patient requires 300 mg/day to achieve an optimal level, but this is very variable and plasma levels are a useful guide. They can be less reliable with other anticonvulsants.

Phenobarbitone	15– 40 mg/l
Sodium valproate	50–100 mg/l
Ethosuximide	40– 80 mg/l
Carbamazepine	8– 12 mg/l

Salicylates

Salicylate in the urine can be detected by Phenistix (Ames) or by a purple colour which occurs when ferric chloride 10% is added dropwise. The colour persists with boiling, unlike that caused by ketone bodies. Serum is positive with Phenistix at salicylate levels of over 900 mg/l. Complex metabolic disturbances occur in salicylate poisoning. In adults and older children a respiratory alkalosis precedes a complex metabolic acidosis, but in young children respiratory alkalosis is unusual. The metabolic acidosis is due to the salicylic acid and also to its effect on fat, protein and carbohydrate metabolism. Ketonaemia, lactic acidosis, hypoglycaemia or hyperglycaemia occur. Blood levels of below 500 mg/l six hours after ingestion indicate mild toxicity and levels of over 750 mg/l are associated with severe toxicity. The blood level should be repeated after 4–6 hours. In rheumatic fever the therapeutic level is 100–300 mg/l and a level of 250 mg/l should be reached, if tolerated, before it is assumed that the drug is ineffective.

Paracetamol

The main danger of poisoning is hepatic necrosis, but renal tubular necrosis may also occur in severe cases. Liver function tests may become abnormal by twelve hours, but maximal disturbance is seen at five days. Four hours after ingestion a paracetamol level of over 200 mg/l indicates probable liver damage and a level of over 500 mg/l is very dangerous. At twelve hours the respective levels are 70 mg/l and 200 mg/l.

Psychotropic Agents

For obvious reasons self-poisoning with these drugs is common. Immediate and skilled supportive care for vital systems is paramount. The removal of unabsorbed drug by gastric aspiration is important and the removal of absorbed drug by diuresis, dialysis and haemoperfusion can be useful. Specific antidotes are helpful in a few situations. With tricyclic and tetracyclic antidepressants there is a particular danger of cardiac arrhythmias and cardiac arrest, so ECG monitoring is vital. Coma and acidosis occur, especially in children.

Serum barbiturate levels can be misleading, as regular takers acquire tolerance. Phenobarbitone levels of over 80 mg/l should be considered dangerous as should levels of over 30 mg/l for the shorter acting drugs, such as amylobarbitone. The therapeutic level for lithium is 0.6–1.5 mmol/l and levels over 2 mmol/l are dangerous. Renal failure, diuretics and fluid depletion can all increase the lithium level.

Alcohol (Ethanol)

The rate of rise of the blood alcohol concentration depends on the total dose, the strength of the solution and associated food intake. After reaching a peak, blood concentrations fall at a rate of about 20 mg per 100 ml per h, but faster in habitual drinkers. Alveolar air concentration is in equilibrium with that of the blood, but the urine concentration is about one-third higher. Intoxicated behaviour may become apparent at levels of between 50 and 150 mg per 100 ml, stupor appears at levels over 300 mg per 100 ml, and above 480 mg per 100 ml there is coma and danger of death. Regular drinkers, however, tolerate much higher levels. Macrocytosis without anaemia may suggest chronic alcoholism and there may be raised serum aminotransferases and γ-GT and a low blood urea.

Iron

A serum level of over 90 μmol/l (500 μg per 100 ml) in a child or of over 145 μmol/l (800 μg per 100 ml) in an adult indicates severe poisoning. Toxicity is also gauged by the excess of iron above the total iron binding capacity (TIBC). Where the TIBC is raised, as in pregnancy, relatively high levels may not be pathological.

Lead

Normal
Heparinized blood
Adults   < 40 μg per 100 ml (< 1.8 μmol/l)
Children   < 30 μg per 100 ml (< 1.45 μmol/l)

The level in exposed workers should be below 60 μg per 100 ml. Haemolytic anaemia with basophilic stippling of the red cells is suggestive. Porphyrin metabolism may be disturbed, with increased urinary excretion of porphobilinogen and coproporphyrins (p. 135). Encephalopathy occurs at levels over 100 μg per 100 ml.

Miscellaneous Therapeutic Concentrations
Clonazepam   15–60 μg/l
Isoniazid   1– 7 mg/l
Procainamide 4–10 mg/l
Theophylline 10–20 mg/l

APPENDIX I

BIBLIOGRAPHY

Clinical Diagnosis

Conn H. F. & Conn R. B. (1980) *Current Diagnosis*, 6th edn. Philadelphia: W. B. Saunders.

Krupp M. A. & Chatton M. J. (1982) *Current Medical Diagnosis and Treatment*. Los Altos, CA: Lange Medical Publications.

Wyngaarden J. B. & Smith L. H. Jr (eds) (1982) *Cecil Textbook of Medicine*, 16th edn. Philadelphia: W. B. Saunders.

These are concise summaries of clinical and laboratory diagnosis.

Methods and Results

Acheson H. W. K. (ed) (1978) *Laboratory, A Manual for the Medical Practitioner*. London: Kluwer Publishing.

Baron D. N., Broughton P. M. G., Cohen M., Lansley, T. S., Lewis S. M. & Shinton N. K. (1974). The use of SI units in reporting results obtained in hospital laboratories *J. Clin. Pathol.*, 27(7): 590–7.

British Medical Association (1981) *Procedures in Practice*. London: British Medical Association. [Articles from Brit. Med. J.]

Hytten F. E. & Lind T. (1973) *Diagnostic Indices in Pregnancy*. Basle: Ciba-Geigy.

Tietz N. W. (ed) (1983) *Clinical Guide to Laboratory Tests*. Philadelphia: W. B. Saunders.

Accounts of available tests, methods and normal results. The supraregional assay service booklet kept in the laboratory will also be found most useful, especially in the field of endocrinology.

Clinical Chemistry

Eastham R. D. (1978) *Biochemical Values in Clinical Medicine*, 6th edn. Bristol: John Wright.

Whitby L. G., Percy-Robb I. W. & Smith A. F. (1980) *Lecture Notes on Clinical Chemistry*, 2nd edn. Oxford: Blackwell Scientific.

Zilva J. F. & Pannall P. R. (1979) *Clinical Chemistry in Diagnosis and Treatment*, 3rd edn. London: Lloyd-Luke (Medical Books).

Bacteriology

Turk D. C. & Porter I. A. (1978) *Short Textbook of Medical Microbiology*, 4th edn. London: Hodder & Stoughton.

Haematology

Dacie J. V. & Lewis S. M. (1975) *Practical Haematology*, 5th edn. Edinburgh: Churchill Livingstone.

Eastham R. D. (1977) *Clinical haematology*, 5th edn. Bristol: John Wright.

Ingram G. I. C., Brozovic M. & Slater N. G. P. (1982) *Bleeding Disorders*, 2nd edn. Oxford: Blackwell Scientific Publications.

Endocrinology

Hall R., Anderson J., Smart G. A. & Besser G. M. (1981) *Fundamentals of Clinical Endocrinology*, 3rd edn. Tunbridge Wells: Pitman Medical.

Ratcliffe J. G. (1981) Hormone assays, *Med. Int.* 6: 231–7.

Paediatrics

Behrman R. & Vaughan V. C. (eds) (1983) *Nelson Textbook of Paediatrics*, 12th edn. Philadelphia: W. B. Saunders.

Wallach J. (1983) *Interpretation of Pediatric Tests*. Boston: Little, Brown.

Electrocardiography

Schamroth L. (1982) *An Introduction to Electrocardiography*, 6th edn. Oxford: Blackwell Scientific.

Radiology

Griffiths H. J. & Sarno R. C. (1979) *Contemporary Radiology*. Philadelphia: W. B. Saunders.

APPENDIX II

UNITS OF MEASUREMENT

Prefixes for decimal multiples and submultiples of units

1000	$= 10^3$	$=$ kilo-(k)
100	$= 10^2$	$=$ hecto-(h)
10	$= 10^1$	$=$ deca-(da)
0.1	$= 10^{-1}$	$=$ deci-(d)
0.01	$= 10^{-2}$	$=$ centi-(c)
0.001	$= 10^{-3}$	$=$ milli-(m)
0.000 001	$= 10^{-6}$	$=$ micro-(μ)
0.000 000 001	$= 10^{-9}$	$=$ nano (n)
0.000 000 000 001	$= 10^{-12}$	$=$ pico-(p)
e.g. 1 microgram	$= 1$ μg	$= 1 \times 10^{-6}$ g

Conversion factors

1 inch	$=$ 2.54 cm
1 pound	$=$ 454 g
1 square foot (ft^2)	$=$ 0.09 square metre (m^2)
1 pint (UK)	$=$ 568 ml
1 pint (US)	$=$ 473 ml

Body surface area

$$S = W^{0.425} \times H^{0.725} \times 71.84$$

$$\log S = \log W \times 0.425 + \log H \times 0.725 + 1.8654$$

where S = surface area (cm^2) = (m$^2 \times 10^4$), W = weight (kg), H = height (cm). Note that nomograms are available to determine S from H and W. Physiological measurements are often adjusted to a standard S of 1.73 m^2. S is more closely related to H than to W.

APPENDIX III

CONVERSION FACTORS, SI TO METRIC UNITS

Bilirubin	μmol/l	× 0.06	= mg/dl
Calcium	mmol/l	× 4	= mg/dl
Cholesterol	mmol/l	× 40	= mg/dl
Cortisol	nmol/l	× 0.035	= μg/dl
Creatinine	μmol/l	× 0.011	= mg/dl
Fat (faecal)	mmol	× 0.3	= g
Glucose	mmol/l	× 18	= mg/dl
Iron	μmol/l	× 5.6	= μg/dl
Phosphorus	mmol/l	× 3	= mg/dl
Triglyceride	mmol/l	× 90	= mg/dl
Urate	mmol/l	× 17	= mg/dl
Urea	mmol/l	× 6	= mg/dl
P_{O_2}	kPa	× 7.5	= mmHg
P_{CO_2}	kPa	× 7.5	= mmHg

Corrections to the nearest 5%.

Conversion equation:

$$\text{Concentration (mg per dl)} = \frac{\text{Concentration (mmol/l)} \times \text{Molecular weight}}{10}$$

INDEX

287